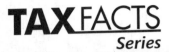

ALL ABOUT
MEDICARE

2007

Hospital Insurance

Medical Insurance

Prescription Drug Insurance

Medigap

Medicaid

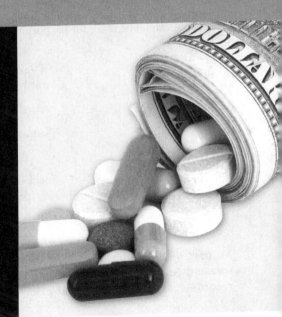

John H. Fenton, J.D., M.S.B.A., Staff Writer

Always Something **NU** to Discover

1-800-543-0874
www.NUCOstore.com

Circular 230 Notice – The content in this publication is not intended or written to be used, and it cannot be used, for the purposes of avoiding U.S. tax penalties.

ISBN 987-0-87218-907-2
ISSN 1044-9426

The National Underwriter Company
P.O. Box 14367, Cincinnati, Ohio 45250-0367

The National Underwriter Company publishes the following Social Security/Medicare publications:

Social Security Manual
All About Medicare
Social Security Slide-O-Scope and Planner
Medicare Planner

TABLE OF CONTENTS

INTRODUCTION

A-1. What is Medicare?

Medicare is a federal health insurance program for persons 65 or older, persons of any age with permanent kidney failure, and certain disabled persons.

Medicare is administered by the Centers for Medicare & Medicaid Services (CMS), a federal agency in the Department of Health and Human Services. Social Security Administration offices across the country take applications for Medicare, collect premiums, and provide general information about the program. Various commercial insurance companies are under contract with CMS to process and pay Medicare claims, and groups of doctors and other health care professionals have contracts to monitor the quality of care delivered to Medicare beneficiaries. CMS also forms partnerships with the thousands of providers of health care services – hospitals, nursing homes, and home health agencies; doctors; suppliers of medical equipment; clinical laboratories; and managed care plans such as health maintenance organizations (HMOs). CMS is located at 7500 Security Boulevard, Baltimore, Maryland 21244.

Medicare consists of Hospital Insurance (Part A), Medical Insurance (Part B), Medicare Advantage (Part C) (formerly known as Medicare+Choice), and Prescription Drug Insurance (Part D).

Hospital Insurance (Part A) provides institutional care, including inpatient hospital care, skilled nursing home care, post-hospital home health care, and, under certain circumstances, hospice care. Part A is financed for the most part by Social Security payroll tax deductions which are deposited in the Federal Hospital Insurance Trust Fund. Medicare beneficiaries also participate in the financing of Part A by paying deductibles, coinsurance, and premiums.

Medical Insurance (Part B) is a voluntary program of health insurance which covers physician's services, outpatient hospital care, physical therapy, ambulance trips, medical equipment, prosthesis, and a number of other services not covered under Part A. It is financed through monthly premiums paid by those who enroll and contributions from the federal government, both of which are deposited into the Federal Supplementary Medical Insurance Trust Fund. The government's share of the cost of Medicare Part B is approximately 75%.

Medicare Advantage (Part C) permits contracts between CMS and a variety of different managed care and fee-for-service organizations. Most Medicare beneficiaries can choose to receive benefits through the original Medicare fee-for-service program or through one of the following Medicare Advantage plans:

- Coordinated care plans, including Health Maintenance Organizations (HMOs), Preferred Provider Organizations (PPOs), and Provider Sponsored Organizations (PSOs). A PSO is defined as a public or private organization, established by health care providers, that provides a substantial proportion of health care items and services directly through affiliated providers who share, directly or indirectly, substantial financial risk.

- Religious fraternal benefit society plans that may restrict enrollment to members of the church, convention or group with which the society is affiliated. Payments to these plans may be adjusted, as appropriate, to take into account the actuarial characteristics and experience of plan enrollees.

- Private fee-for-service plans that reimburse providers on a fee-for-service basis, and are authorized to charge enrolled beneficiaries up to 115% of the plan's payment schedule (which may be different from the Medicare fee schedule).

The Department of Health and Human Services contracts with private insurance companies for the processing of payments to patients and health care providers. These private insurance companies are called fiscal intermediaries under Part A and are selected by the health care providers. Under Part B, these private insurance companies are called carriers and are selected by the Department of Health and Human Services.

Medicare Prescription Drug Insurance (Part D) was added to Medicare by the Medicare Prescription Drug, Improvement, and Modernization Act of 2003. In exchange for a monthly premium, Medicare Part D participants receive limited coverage for prescription drug benefits up to a catastrophic coverage threshold, above which Part D will cover roughly 95% of prescription drug costs. The Medicare Part D prescription drug program was effective beginning January 1, 2006.

A-2. What federal agency administers Medicare?

The Centers for Medicare & Medicaid Services (CMS), whose central office is in Baltimore, Maryland, directs the Medicare and Medicaid programs. The Social Security Administration processes Medicare applications and claims, but it does not set Medicare policy. CMS sets the standards that hospitals, skilled nursing facilities, home health agencies, and hospices must meet in order to be certified as qualified providers of services. It also establishes the reimbursement rate of all covered services.

A-3. In general, what is the Hospital Insurance (Part A) protection provided by Medicare?

Persons protected have benefits paid for certain hospital and related health care services when they incur expenses for such services.

A person entitled to Social Security monthly benefits or a qualified railroad retirement beneficiary is automatically entitled to Hospital Insurance protection beginning with the first day of the month of attainment of age 65. An individual who is insured for monthly benefits need not actually file to receive the benefits. Under limited circumstances, services furnished in Canada or Mexico, or in some cases in the Caribbean, or aboard ship in United States territorial waters, may be paid by Medicare, but otherwise, services furnished outside the United States are not paid for by Hospital Insurance.

Medicare is the secondary payer if a person is covered by an employer group health insurance plan, is entitled to veterans benefits, workers' compensation, or black lung benefits. Medicare is also the secondary payer if no-fault insurance or liability insurance (such as automobile insurance) is available as the primary payer. Although Medicare is sometimes the secondary payer when liability insurance is available, Medicare may make a conditional payment if it receives a claim for services covered by liability insurance. In these cases, Medicare recovers its conditional payment from the settlement amount when the liability settlement is reached.

Medicare is the secondary payer during a period (generally 30 months) for individuals who have Medicare solely on the basis of their end-stage renal disease, if they have employer group health plan coverage themselves or through a family member.

A-4. In general, what is the Medical Insurance (Part B) protection provided by Medicare?

Persons protected have benefits paid for certain physicians' services (including surgery), home health services (other than post-hospital home health services), clinical laboratory services, durable medical equipment, and some other items and services not covered by Hospital Insurance (Part A) protection.

Medical Insurance (Part B) protection is financed through monthly premiums paid by each person who enrolls (or by the state where the person is enrolled under a federal-state agreement) and through contributions appropriated from federal general revenues. Beginning in 2007, the premium for Part B varies according to a person's income. The standard monthly premium for Part B coverage beginning January 1, 2007 is $93.50. Those with higher incomes may pay as much as $161.40 in 2007. For a detailed explanation of the Part B premiums, see C-7.

A-5. Who can provide services or supplies under Medicare?

Health care organizations and professionals providing services to Medicare beneficiaries must meet all licensing requirements of state or local health authorities. The organizations and persons listed below also must meet additional Medicare certification requirements before payments can be made for their services:

- Hospitals

- Skilled nursing facilities

- Home health agencies

- Hospice programs

- Independent diagnostic laboratories and organizations providing X-ray services

- Organizations providing outpatient physical therapy and speech pathology services

- Facilities providing outpatient rehabilitation facilities

- Ambulance firms

- Chiropractors

3

- Independent physical therapists (those who furnish services in the patient's home or in their offices)

- Facilities providing kidney dialysis or transplant services

- Rural health clinics

All hospitals, skilled nursing facilities, and home health agencies participating in the Medicare program must comply with Title VI of the Civil Rights Act, which prohibits discrimination because of race, color, creed, or national origin.

Medicare does not pay for care received from a hospital, skilled nursing facility, home health agency, or hospice that is not certified to participate in the program. These providers are referred to as non-participating. But Hospital Insurance can help pay for care in a qualified non-participating hospital if (1) the patient is admitted to the non-participating hospital for emergency treatment, and (2) the non-participating hospital is the closest one that is equipped to handle the emergency. Under Medicare, emergency treatment means treatment that is immediately necessary to prevent death or serious impairment to health.

If the non-participating hospital elects to submit the claim for Medicare payment, Medicare will pay the hospital directly except for any deductible or coinsurance amounts. If the hospital does not submit the claim, the patient may submit the claim and receive payment. In this case, the patient would reimburse the hospital.

A-6. In general, what benefits are provided under the Hospital Insurance (Part A) program?

The program, which is compulsory, provides the following benefits for persons age 65 or older and persons receiving Social Security disability benefits for 24 months or more:

- The cost of inpatient hospital care for up to 90 days in each benefit period (for 2007, the patient pays a deductible amount of $992 for the first 60 days plus $248 a day for each day in excess of 60). There are also 60 non-renewable lifetime reserve days with coinsurance of $496 a day in 2007.

- The cost of post-hospital skilled nursing facility care for up to 100 days in each benefit period (the patient pays $124.00 a day in 2007 after the first 20 days).

- The cost of 100 post-hospital or post-skilled nursing facility home health service visits in a spell of illness made under a plan of treatment established by a physician, except that there is 20% cost-sharing payable by the patient for durable medical equipment (other than the purchase of certain used items). Additional coverage for home health care services which do not meet the Part A coverage criteria and visit limitations may be available under Medical Insurance (Part B). (See A-8.)

- The cost of hospice care for terminally ill patients.

For a detailed explanation of these benefits, see SECTION B.

A-7. In general, what benefits are payable under Medical Insurance (Part B)?

Medical Insurance (Part B) is offered to almost all persons age 65 or over on a voluntary basis. In addition, the program is offered to all disabled Social Security and Railroad Retirement beneficiaries who have received disability benefits for at least 24 months. For 2007, there is an annual deductible of $131, paid by the patient. Since 2005, this annual deductible is adjusted to reflect increases in Medicare Part B costs. Medical Insurance pays 80% of the approved charges above the deductible for the following services:

- Physicians' and surgeons' services, whether furnished in a hospital, clinic, office, home, or elsewhere, excluding routine or yearly physical exams.

- A one-time initial wellness physical in within 6 months of enrolling in Medical Insurance (Part B).

- Screening blood tests for early detection of cardiovascular disease.

- Diabetes screening tests for those at risk of getting diabetes.

- Home health care visits, if not covered under Hospital Insurance (Part A) (but with no cost-sharing except for durable medical equipment, other than the purchase of certain used items). In the past, few home health care visits were covered under Medical Insurance (Part B) but this has changed because of the creation of separate Hospital Insurance and Medical Insurance home health benefits in 1998. (See A-8.)

- Outpatient hospital services for the diagnosis or treatment of an illness or injury.

- Diagnostic x-ray tests (including certain portable X-ray services in the home), diagnostic laboratory tests, and other diagnostic tests (no cost-sharing).

- Outpatient physical therapy and outpatient speech-language pathology services furnished by participating hospitals, skilled nursing facilities, home health agencies, outpatient therapy clinics, or by others under arrangements with and under the supervision of such organizations.

- Outpatient physical therapy services and outpatient speech-language pathology services provided in a hospital or skilled nursing facility to its inpatients who have exhausted their inpatient days, or are otherwise not entitled to Hospital Insurance benefits.

- Outpatient physical therapy services and occupational therapy services furnished by a licensed, independently practicing physical therapist or occupational therapist in his or her office or the patient's home, provided the patient is under the care of a physician.

- Rural health clinic services and federally qualified health center services.

- Prosthetic devices (other than dental) which replace all or part of a covered body part, including replacement of such devices.

- Home dialysis supplies and equipment, self-care home dialysis support services, and institutional dialysis and supplies.

- Chiropractor's treatment by manual manipulation of the spine to correct a subluxation of the spine. But the cost of the chiropractor's X-ray, if any, is excluded.

- Podiatrist's services (excluding the treatment of flat foot conditions, subluxations of the foot, and routine foot care that does not require treatment by a podiatrist or physician).

- Leg, arm, back, and neck braces, and artificial legs, arms, and eyes, including replacements where necessary because of a change in the patient's condition.

- Rental or purchase of durable medical equipment.

- X-ray, radium, and radioactive isotope therapy, including materials and services of technicians.

- Surgical dressings, and splints, casts, and other devices for reduction of fractures and dislocations.

- Ambulance services, under certain circumstances.

- Blood clotting factors for hemophilia patients and items related to its administration.

- Hospital services incident to a physician's services to an outpatient (including drugs and biologicals which cannot be self-administered).

- Antigens prepared by a physician for a particular patient.

- Annual flu shot (no cost-sharing).

- Pneumococcal vaccine and its administration (no cost-sharing).

- Hepatitis B vaccine and its administration (if beneficiary considered at high or intermediate risk of contracting disease).

- Certified nurse-midwife services.

- Partial hospitalization services provided by a community mental health center or hospital outpatient department.

- Screening pap smear and pelvic exams.

- Prostate cancer screening tests.

- Annual screening mammography for all women age 40 and over (the Part B deductible is waived).

- Colorectal cancer screening.

- Diabetes monitoring and self-management benefits.

- Bone mass measurements.

- The cost of an injectable drug for the treatment of a bone fracture related to post-menopausal osteoporosis.

- Eyeglasses following cataract surgery.

- Services of nurse practitioners and clinical nurse specialists in rural areas for the services they are authorized to perform under state law and regulations.

- Oral cancer drugs if they are the same chemical entity as those administered intravenously and currently covered. Off-label cancer drugs are covered in some cases.

- Necessary medical supplies.

- Immunosuppressive drug therapy.

- Lung and heart-lung, liver and kidney transplants under certain circumstances.

The cost of psychiatric treatment outside a hospital for mental, psychoneurotic, and personality disorders is covered. But coinsurance is usually 50% instead of 20%.

For a detailed explanation of these benefits, see SECTION C.

A-8. What is the difference between home health care coverage under Hospital Insurance and Medical Insurance?

Home health services unassociated with a hospital or skilled nursing facility stay were gradually transferred from Part A to Part B. Medicare Part A continues to cover the first 100 visits in a spell of illness following a 3-day hospital stay or a skilled nursing facility stay.

The transfer was phased in over a period of seven years between 1998 and 2004. Beginning in 2004, Part A covers only post-institutional home health services for up to 100 visits during a home health spell of illness, except for those persons with Part A coverage only who will be covered for services without regard to the post-institutional limitation.

A-9. Is there any overall limit to the benefits a person can receive under Medicare?

Under Hospital Insurance (Part A), benefits begin anew in each benefit period. In addition, there are no dollar limits under Medical Insurance (Part B) except for psychiatric care and independent physical and occupational therapy. Under Hospital Insurance, care in a psychiatric hospital is subject to a lifetime limit of 190 days. (The time a patient has spent in a hospital for psychiatric care immediately prior to becoming eligible for Medicare counts against the special 150-day limit in the first hospitalization period, but not against the 190-day lifetime limit.)

Separate calendar year caps ($1,780 in 2007) on coverage of independent occupational therapy and physical and speech therapy services returned January 1, 2006. The annual limitation was initially enacted for 1999, but Congress granted and then extended a moratorium on implementation through the end of 2002. Implementation was further delayed by administration decision until September 1, 2003. The limitation was then eliminated effective December 7, 2003. The Medicare Prescription Drug, Improvement, and Modernization Act of 2003 eliminated the annual limit through the end of 2005. In the Deficit Reduction Act of 2005, Congress added a provision for the Secretary of Health and Human Services to make an exception to the annual limit if the provision of additional services is "medically necessary." The exceptions process allows for specific diagnoses and procedures to receive Medicare coverage even after a beneficiary has met their therapy cap for the year. Alternatively, a provider can request an exception if the particular problem to be treated is not automatically covered under the given exceptions. This exceptions process was scheduled to end January 1, 2007, but has been extended through December 31, 2007.

Medicare may limit benefit payments for services for which other third party insurance programs (e.g., workers' compensation, automobile or liability insurance, and employer health plans) may ultimately be liable. The Spending Reduction Act of 1984 establishes the statutory right of Medicare to:(1) bring an action against any entity that would be primarily responsible for payment with respect to the item or service, (2) bring an action against any entity (including any physician or provider) that has been paid with respect to the item or service, and (3) join or intervene in an action against a third party.

A-10. When do Medicare benefits become available?

Medicare benefits become available at the beginning of the month in which an individual reaches age 65. This is true even if the individual is still working. Medicare benefits are also available after an individual has been receiving Social Security disability benefits for two years or has end-stage renal disease requiring renal dialysis or a kidney transplant.

A-11. What is a Medicare card?

A Medicare card is issued after a person becomes eligible for Medicare benefits. The card shows the person's coverage (Hospital Insurance, Medical Insurance, or both) and the date protection started. The card also shows the person's health insurance claim number. The claim number usually has nine digits and one or two letters. On some cards, there will be another number after the letter. The full claim number must always be included on all Medicare claims and correspondence. When a husband and wife both have Medicare, each receives a separate card and claim number. Each spouse must use the exact name and claim number shown on his or her card.

Important points to remember:

- The patient should always show the Medicare card when receiving services that Medicare can help pay for.

- The patient should always write the health insurance claim number (including any letters) on all checks for Medicare premium payments or any correspondence about Medicare. Also, the patient should have the Medicare card available when making a telephone inquiry.

- The patient should carry the card whenever away from home. If it is lost, immediately ask a representative at any Social Security office for a new one.

- The patient should use the Medicare card only after the effective date shown on the card.

- Medicare cards made of metal or plastic, which are sold by some manufacturers, are not a substitute for the officially issued Medicare card.

- Never permit someone else to use your Medicare card.

A-12. What care is not covered under Medicare?

Medicare does not cover custodial care when that is the only kind of care the patient needs.

Care is considered custodial when it is primarily for the purpose of helping with daily living or meeting personal needs and could be provided safely and reasonably by persons without professional skills or training. Much of the care provided in nursing homes to people with chronic, long-term illnesses or disabilities is considered custodial care. For example, custodial care includes help in walking, getting in and out of bed, bathing, dressing, eating, and taking medicine. Even if an individual is in a participating hospital or skilled nursing facility or the individual is receiving care from a participating home health agency, Medicare does not cover the stay if the patient needs only custodial care.

Medicare does not pay for services that are not reasonable and necessary for the diagnosis or treatment of an illness or injury. These services include drugs or devices that have not been approved by the Food and Drug Administration (FDA); medical procedures and services performed using drugs or devices not approved by FDA; and services, including drugs or devices, not considered safe and effective because they are experimental or investigational. In addition, Medicare does not pay for most outpatient prescription drugs (except under Medicare Part D), routine or annual physical exams, most dental care and dentures, routine foot care, routine eye care, hearing aids and cosmetic surgery.

If a doctor places an individual in a hospital or skilled nursing facility when the kind of care the individual needs could be provided elsewhere, the individual's stay will not be considered reasonable and necessary, and Medicare will not pay for it. If an individual stays in a hospital or skilled nursing facility longer than necessary, Medicare payments will end when inpatient care is no longer reasonable or necessary.

If a doctor (or other practitioner) comes to treat a person or that person visits the doctor for treatment more often than is medically necessary, Medicare will not pay for the "extra" visits.

Medicare will not pay for services performed by immediate relatives or members of a patient's household. Medicare also will not pay for services paid for by another government program.

Doctors cannot make self-referrals for certain designated health services. Designated health services include (1) clinical laboratory services, (2) physical therapy services, (3) occupational therapy services, (4) radiology services, including MRI, CAT scans, and ultrasound services, (5) radiation therapy services and supplies, (6) durable medical equipment and supplies, (7) parenteral and enteral nutrients, equipment, and supplies, (8) prosthetics, orthotics, and prosthetic devices and supplies, (9) home health services, (10) outpatient prescription drugs, and (11) inpatient and outpatient hospital services.

The law prohibits a doctor who has a financial relationship with an entity from referring Medicare patients to that entity to receive a designated health service. The prohibition also applies if a doctor's immediate family member has a financial relationship with the entity. A financial relationship can exist as an ownership or investment interest in *or* a compensation arrangement with an entity. The law is triggered by the mere fact that a financial relationship exists; it does not matter what the doctor intends when making a referral.

An entity cannot bill Medicare, Medicaid, the beneficiary, or anyone else for a designated health service furnished to a Medicare patient under a prohibited referral. If a person collects any amount for services billed in violation of the law, a refund must be made. A person can be subject to a civil money penalty or exclusion from Medicare if that person (1) presents or causes to be presented a claim to Medicare or bill to any individual, third party payer, or other entity for any designated health service the person knows or should know was furnished as the result of a prohibited referral, or (2) fails to make a timely refund.

Under Medicare law a person will not be held responsible for payment of the cost of certain health care services for which the person was denied Medicare payment if the person did not know or could not reasonably be expected to know that the services were not covered by Medicare. This provision is often referred to as a "Waiver of Liability." The waiver provision applies only when the care was denied because it was one of the following: (1) custodial care, (2) not reasonable or necessary under Medicare program standards for diagnosis or treatment, (3) for home health services, the patient was not homebound or not receiving skilled nursing care on an intermittent basis, or (4) the only reason for the denial is that, in error, the patient was placed in a skilled nursing facility bed that was not approved by Medicare.

Also, the limitation of liability provision does not apply to Medical Insurance services provided by a non-participating physician or supplier who did not accept assignment of the claim. However, in certain situations Medicare will protect the patient from paying for services provided by a non-participating physician on a non-assigned basis that are denied as "not reasonable and necessary." If a physician knows or should know that Medicare will not pay for a particular service as "not reasonable and necessary," the physician must give the patient written notice – before performing the service – of the reasons why he believes Medicare will not pay. The physician must get the patient's written agreement to pay for the services. If the patient does not receive this notice, he is not required to pay for the service. If the patient pays for the service, but did not receive a notice, he may be entitled to a refund.

A-13. What are quality improvement organizations?

Quality Improvement Organizations (QIOs) are groups of practicing doctors and other health care professionals who are paid by the federal government to review the care given to Medicare patients. Each state has a QIO that decides, for Medicare payment purposes, whether care is reasonable, necessary, and provided in the most appropriate setting. QIOs also decide whether care meets the standards of quality generally accepted by the medical profession. QIOs have the authority to deny payments if care is not medically necessary or not delivered in the most appropriate setting.

QIOs investigate individual patient complaints about the quality of care and respond to (1) requests for review of notices of noncoverage issued by hospitals to beneficiaries, and (2) requests for reconsideration of QIO decisions by beneficiaries, physicians, and hospitals.

The QIO will tell the patient in writing if the service received was not covered by Medicare.

If a patient is admitted to a Medicare-participating hospital, the patient will receive *An Important Message From Medicare*, which explains the patient's rights as a hospital patient and provides the name, address and phone number of the QIO in the patient's state.

If a patient believes he has been improperly refused admission to a hospital, forced to leave a hospital too soon, or denied coverage of a medical procedure or treatment, the patient should ask for a written explanation of the decision. This written notice must fully explain how the patient can appeal the decision, and it must give the patient the name, address and phone number of the QIO where an appeal or request for review can be submitted.

If a patient disagrees with the decision of a QIO, the patient can appeal by requesting a reconsideration. Then, if the patient disagrees with the QIO's reconsideration decision and the amount in question is $200 or more, the patient can request a hearing by an Administrative Law Judge. Cases involving $2,000 or more can eventually be appealed to a federal court.

Appeals of decisions on all other services covered under Hospital Insurance (skilled nursing facility care, home health care, hospice services, and some inpatient hospital matters not handled by QIOs) are handled by Medicare intermediaries.

For a detailed explanation of the appeals process, see SECTION F.

A-14. When should a person use the Medicare fraud and abuse hotline?

If a person has reason to believe that a doctor, hospital, or other provider of health care services is performing unnecessary or inappropriate services, or is billing Medicare for services not received, the person should report this information to the Medicare carrier or intermediary that handles his claims.

If the Medicare carrier or intermediary does not respond to a person's report of Medicare fraud or abuse, the person may call the Centers for Medicare & Medicaid Services (CMS) hotline at 1-800-447-8477 (1-800-HHS-TIPS). Be prepared to tell (1) the exact nature of the suspected wrongdoing, the date it occurred, and the name and address of the party involved, (2) the name and location of the Medicare intermediary or carrier the person reported it to, and when it was reported, and (3) the name of any intermediary or carrier employee the person spoke with and what advice the intermediary or carrier gave to the person.

The federal government contracts with private insurance organizations called *intermediaries* and *carriers* to process claims and make Medicare payments. Intermediaries handle inpatient and outpatient claims submitted on the patient's behalf to hospitals, skilled nursing facilities, home health agencies, hospices and certain other providers of services under Hospital Insurance (Part A). Carriers handle claims for services by doctors and suppliers covered under Medical Insurance (Part B). If a patient has questions about Medical Insurance claims, he should contact the Medicare carrier in his state.

Individuals are encouraged to report information on individuals and organizations engaged in acts or omissions that constitute grounds for sanction under the Social Security Act, or who have engaged in fraud and abuse against the Medicare program. If an individual reports information that serves as the basis for the collection of $100 or more, the CMS may pay a portion of the amount collected to the individual. Individuals are also encouraged to submit suggestions on methods to improve the efficiency of the Medicare program. If the suggestion is adopted and savings to the program result, a payment may be made to the individual of an amount the CMS considers appropriate.

A-15. Should a person receive Medicare benefits through the fee-for-service system or through a Medicare Advantage managed care plan?

A person living in an area serviced by a managed care plan has a choice between the fee-for-service system or a managed care plan. If a person chooses fee-for-service, he can go to almost any doctor, hospital or other health care provider he wants to. Generally, a fee is charged each time a service is used. Medicare pays its share of the bill. The patient is responsible for paying the balance and may obtain a Medicare Supplemental Insurance (Medigap) policy to cover or help defray the patient's share of these charges. See SECTION F on Medigap insurance.

In managed care, a person usually must receive all of his care from the doctors, hospitals, and other health care providers that are part of the plan, except in emergencies. Depending on the plan, the patient may pay a monthly premium and a copayment each time he goes to the doctor or uses other services. The premiums and copayments vary from plan to plan and may change each year.

Regardless of whether a person chooses fee-for-service or managed care, he retains all of his Medicare benefits, protections and appeal rights. See SECTION D for a detailed description of Medicare Advantage.

PART A:
HOSPITAL INSURANCE

ELIGIBILITY

B-1. Who is eligible for benefits under Hospital Insurance?

All persons age 65 and over who are entitled to monthly Social Security cash benefits (or would be entitled except that an application for cash benefits has not been filed), or monthly cash benefits under Railroad Retirement programs (whether retired or not), are eligible for benefits.

Persons age 65 and over can receive Medicare benefits even if they continue to work. Enrollment in the program while working will not affect the amount of future Social Security benefits.

A dependent or survivor of a person entitled to Hospital Insurance benefits, or a dependent of a person under age 65 who is entitled to retirement or disability benefits, is also eligible for Hospital Insurance (Part A) benefits if the dependent or survivor is at least 65 years old. For example, a woman age 65 or over who is entitled to a spouse's or widow's Social Security benefit is eligible for benefits under Hospital Insurance.

A Social Security disability beneficiary is covered under Medicare after entitlement to disability benefits for 24 months or more. Those covered include disabled workers at any age, disabled widows and widowers age 50 or over, beneficiaries age 18 or older who receive benefits because of disability beginning before age 22, and disabled qualified railroad retirement annuitants. Medicare coverage is automatic. No application is required.

A person who becomes re-entitled to disability benefits within five years after the end of a previous period of entitlement (within seven years in the case of disabled widows or widowers and disabled children) is automatically eligible for Medicare coverage without the need to wait another 24 months. However, and further, if the previous period of disability ends on or after March 1, 1988, he is covered under Medicare without again needing to meet the 24 month waiting period requirement, regardless of not meeting the five year (or seven year) requirement, if the current impairment is the same as (or directly related to) that in the previous period of disability.

Coverage will continue for 24 months after an individual is no longer entitled to receive disability payments because he has returned to work, provided he was considered disabled on or after December 10, 1980, and the disabling condition continues.

B-2. What are the special eligibility rules for persons with end-stage renal disease?

Insured workers (and their dependents) with end-stage renal disease who require renal dialysis or a kidney transplant are deemed disabled for Medicare coverage purposes even if they are working. Coverage can begin with the first day of the third month after

13

the month dialysis treatments begin. This three-month waiting period is waived if the individual participates in a self-care dialysis training course during the waiting period.

Medicare coverage based on a kidney transplant begins with the month of the transplant or with either of the two preceding months if the patient was hospitalized during either of those months for procedures preliminary to the transplant. If entitlement could be based on more than one of the factors, the earliest date is used.

Coverage is provided under Medicare for the self-administration of erythropoietin for home renal dialysis patients.

Medicare is the secondary payer during a period (generally 30 months) for individuals who have Medicare solely on the basis of their end-stage renal disease, if they have employer group health plan coverage themselves or through a family member. During this period, if an employer plan pays less than the provider's charges, then Medicare may supplement the plan's payments. (See B-4.)

B-3. What are the special eligibility rules for government employees?

Federal employees who were not covered under Social Security (temporary workers have been covered since 1951) began paying the Hospital Insurance (HI) portion of Social Security tax in 1983. Those covered under Social Security, such as virtually all hired after 1983, pay the HI tax as well as the Social Security Old-Age, Survivors, and Disability Insurance (OASDI) tax. A transitional provision provides credit for retroactive hospital quarters of coverage for federal employees who were employed before 1983 and also on January 1, 1983.

State and local government employees hired after March 31, 1986, are covered under Medicare coverage and tax provisions. A person who was performing substantial and regular service for a state or local government before April 1, 1986, is not covered provided he was a bona fide employee on March 31, 1986, and the employment relationship was not entered into in order to meet the requirements for exemptions from coverage.

State or local government employees whose employment is terminated after March 31, 1986, are covered under Medicare if they are later rehired.

Beginning after June 30, 1991, state and local government workers who are not covered by a retirement system in conjunction with their employment, and who are not already subject to the HI tax, are also automatically covered and must pay the tax. A retirement system is defined as a pension, annuity, retirement, or similar fund or system established by a state or by a political subdivision of a state.

Individuals are not automatically covered under Medicare if employed by a state or local government

(1) to relieve them of unemployment;

(2) in a hospital, home, or institution where they are inmates or patients;

(3) on a temporary basis because of an emergency such as a storm, earthquake, flood, fire or snow;

(4) if the individuals qualify as interns, student nurses or other student employees of District of Columbia government hospitals, unless the individuals are medical or dental interns or medical or dental residents in training.

State governments may voluntarily enter into agreements to extend Medicare coverage to employees not covered under the rules above.

B-4. When is Medicare considered a secondary payer?

There are limitations on Medicare payments for services covered under group health plans. Medicare is secondary payer, under specified conditions, for services covered under any of the following:

- Group health plans of employers that employ at least 20 employees and that cover Medicare beneficiaries age 65 or older who are covered under the plan by virtue of the individual's current employment status with an employer or the current employment status of a spouse of any age.

- Group health plans (without regard to the number of individuals employed and irrespective of current employment status) that cover individuals who have end stage renal disease. Generally, group health plans are always primary payers throughout the first 30 months of end stage renal disease based on Medicare eligibility or entitlement.

- Large group health plans (that is, plans of employers that employ at least 100 employees) that cover Medicare beneficiaries who are under age 65, entitled to Medicare on the basis of disability, and covered under the plan by virtue of the individual's or a family member's current employment status with an employer.

Group health plans and large group health plans may not take into account that the individuals described above are entitled to Medicare on the basis of age or disability, or eligible for, or entitled to Medicare on the basis of end stage renal disease. Group health plans of employers of 20 or more employees must provide to any employee or spouse age 65 or older the same benefits, under the same conditions, that it provides to employees and spouses under 65. The requirement applies regardless of whether the individual or spouse 65 or older is entitled to Medicare. Group health plans may not differentiate in the benefits they provide between individuals who have end stage renal disease and other individuals covered under the plan on the basis of the existence of end stage renal disease, the need for renal dialysis, or in any other manner.

A "group health plan" means any arrangement made by one or more employers or employee organizations to provide health care directly or through other methods such as insurance or reimbursement, to current or former employees, the employer, others associated or formerly associated with the employer in a business relationship, or their families, that

(1) is of, or contributed to by, one or more employers or employee organizations;

(2) involves more than one employer or employee organization, provides for common administration; and

(3) provides substantially the same benefits or the same benefit options to all those enrolled under the arrangement.

Group health plans include self-insured plans, plans of governmental entities (federal, state, and local), and employee organization plans (union plans, employee health and welfare funds, or other employee organization plans). Group health plans also include employee-pay-all plans, which are plans under the auspices of one or more employers or employee organizations but which receive no financial contributions from them. Not included in the definition of group health plans are plans that are unavailable to employees; for example, a plan only for self-employed persons.

A large group health plan means a group health plan that covers employees of either

- a single employer or employee organization that employed at least 100 full-time or part-time employees on 50% or more of its regular business days during the previous calendar year, or

- two or more employers, or employee organizations, at least one of which employed at least 100 full-time or part-time employees on 50% or more of its regular business days during the previous calendar year.

An employer or insurer is prohibited from offering Medicare beneficiaries financial or other benefits as incentives not to enroll in, or to terminate enrollment in, a group health plan that is, or would be, primary to Medicare. The prohibition precludes offering to Medicare beneficiaries an alternative to the employer primary plan (for example, coverage of prescription drugs) unless the beneficiary has primary coverage other than Medicare. An example would be primary coverage through his own or a spouse's employer.

Actions by group health plans or large group health plans that constitute "taking into account" that an individual is entitled to Medicare on the basis of end stage renal disease, age, or disability (or eligible on the basis of end stage renal disease) include, but are not limited to, the following:

- failure to pay primary benefits as required

- offering coverage that is secondary to Medicare to individuals entitled to Medicare

- terminating coverage because the individual has become entitled to Medicare, except as permitted under COBRA continuation coverage provisions

- in the case of a large group health plan, denying or terminating coverage because an individual is entitled to Medicare on the basis of disability without denying or terminating coverage for similarly situated individuals who are not entitled to Medicare on the basis of disability

- imposing limitations on benefits for a Medicare entitled individual that do not apply to others enrolled in the plan, such as providing less comprehensive health care coverage, excluding benefits, reducing benefits, charging higher deductibles or coinsurance, providing for lower annual or lifetime benefit limits, or more restrictive pre-existing illness limitations

- charging a Medicare entitled individual higher premiums

- requiring a Medicare entitled individual to wait longer for coverage to begin

- paying providers and suppliers no more than the Medicare payment rate for services furnished to a Medicare beneficiary but making payments at a higher rate for the same services to an enrollee who is not entitled to Medicare

- providing misleading or incomplete information that would have the effect of inducing a Medicare entitled individual to reject the employer plan, thereby making Medicare the primary payer. An example of this would be informing the beneficiary of the right to accept or reject the employer plan but failing to inform the individual that, if he rejects the plan, the plan will not be permitted to provide or pay for secondary benefits

- including in its health insurance cards, claims forms, or brochures distributed to beneficiaries, providers, and suppliers, instructions to bill Medicare first for services furnished to Medicare beneficiaries without stipulating that such action may be taken only when Medicare is the primary payer

- refusing to enroll an individual for whom Medicare would be secondary payer, when enrollment is available to similarly situated individuals for whom Medicare would not be secondary payer

If a group health plan or large group health plan makes benefit distinctions among various categories of individuals (distinctions unrelated to the fact that the individual is disabled), the group health plan or large group health plan may make the same distinctions among the same categories of individuals entitled to Medicare whose plan coverage is based on current employment status. For example, if a group health plan or large group health plan does not offer coverage to employees who have worked less than one year and who are *not* entitled to Medicare on the basis of disability or age, the group health plan or large group health plan is not required to offer coverage to employees who have worked less than one year and who *are* entitled to Medicare on the basis of disability or age.

A group health plan or large group health plan may pay benefits secondary to Medicare for an aged or disabled beneficiary who has current employment status if the plan coverage is COBRA continuation coverage because of reduced hours of work. Medicare is primary payer for this beneficiary because, although he has current employment status, the group health plan coverage is by virtue of the COBRA law rather than by virtue of the current employment status.

Aged Beneficiaries and Spouses

Medicare benefits are secondary to benefits payable by a group health plan for services furnished during any month in which the individual is age 65 or older, eligible for Medicare Part A, and meets one of the following conditions:

(1) The individual is covered under a group health plan of an employer that has at least 20 employees (including a multi-employer plan in which at least one of the participating employers meets that condition), and coverage under the plan is by virtue of the individual's current employment status.

(2) The individual is the aged spouse (including a divorced or common-law spouse) of an individual (of any age) who is covered under a group health plan by virtue of the individual's current employment status.

Disabled Beneficiaries

Medicare benefits are secondary to benefits payable by a large group health plan for services furnished during any month in which the individual (1) is entitled to Medicare Part A benefits on the basis of disability, (2) is covered under a large group health plan, and (3) has large group health plan coverage by virtue of his own or a family member's current employment status.

Medicare becomes primary if the services are (1) furnished to Medicare beneficiaries who have declined to enroll in the group health plan, (2) not covered under the plan for the disabled individual or similarly situated individuals, (3) covered under the plan but not available to particular disabled individuals because they have exhausted their benefits under the plan, (4) furnished to individuals whose COBRA continuation coverage has been terminated because of the individual's Medicare entitlement, or (5) covered under COBRA continuation coverage notwithstanding the individual's Medicare entitlement.

End Stage Renal Disease

A group health plan may not take into account that an individual is eligible for or entitled to Medicare benefits on the basis of end stage renal disease. An individual who has end stage renal disease but who has not filed an application for entitlement to Medicare on that basis is eligible for Medicare based on end stage renal disease. A group health plan may not differentiate in the benefits it provides between individuals who have end stage renal disease and others enrolled in the plan, on the basis of the existence of end stage renal disease, or in any other manner.

Generally, Medicare is secondary payer during the first 30 months of end stage renal disease-based eligibility or entitlement. Medicare becomes primary after the 30th month of end stage renal disease-based eligibility or entitlement.

Examples of group health plan actions that constitute differentiation in plan benefits (and that may constitute "taking into account" Medicare eligibility or entitlement) include

- terminating coverage of the individuals with end stage renal disease, when there is no basis for such termination unrelated to end stage renal disease that would result in termination for individuals who do not have end stage renal disease

- imposing on persons who have end stage renal disease, but not on others enrolled in the plan, benefit limitations such as less comprehensive health plan coverage, reductions in benefits, exclusions of benefits, a higher deductible or coinsurance, a longer waiting period, a lower annual or lifetime benefit limit, or more restrictive pre-existing illness limitations

- charging individuals with end stage renal disease higher premiums

- paying providers and suppliers less for services furnished to individuals who have end stage renal disease, such as paying 80% of the Medicare rate for renal dialysis

- failure to cover routine maintenance dialysis or kidney transplants, when a plan covers other dialysis services or other organ transplants

Other Secondary Payer Rules

An employee may reject the employer's plan and retain Medicare as the primary payer, but regulations prevent employers from offering a health plan or option designed to induce the employee to reject the employer's plan and retain Medicare as primary payer.

For persons who are not eligible for Social Security or Railroad Retirement benefits, see B-5.

Medicare is also the secondary payer

(1) when medical care can be paid for under no-fault insurance or liability insurance (including automobile insurance),

(2) if the individual is entitled to veterans benefits,

(3) if the individual is entitled to black lung benefits, or

(4) if the individual is covered by workers' compensation.

Although Medicare is sometimes the secondary payer when liability insurance is available, Medicare may make a conditional payment if it receives a claim for services covered by liability insurance. In these cases, Medicare recovers its conditional payment from the settlement amount when the liability settlement is reached.

A third party payer must give notice to Medicare if it learns that Medicare has made a primary payment in a situation where the third party payer made or should have made the primary payment. A third party payer is considered to learn that Medicare has made a primary payment when the third party payer receives information that Medicare had made a primary payment, or when it receives information sufficient to draw the conclusion that Medicare has made a primary payment.

Example. The third party payer has received a copy of an Explanation of Medicare Benefits form, and the form shows that Medicare has made a primary payment for services for which the third party has made, or ought to have made, primary payment.

Example. A beneficiary for whom Medicare should be secondary payer states in correspondence provided to the third party payer that Medicare has made primary payment for a given item or service for which the beneficiary has primary coverage under the third party payer's plan.

Example. A beneficiary who is eligible for Medicare files a claim for primary payment with a third party payer, the claim is denied, the beneficiary appeals, and the denial is reversed. (The third party payer should assume that Medicare made a conditional primary payment in the interim.)

The Centers for Medicare & Medicaid Services must mail questionnaires to individuals, before they become entitled to benefits under Hospital Insurance (Part A) or enroll in Medical Insurance (Part B), to determine whether they are covered under a primary plan. Payments will not be denied for covered services solely on the grounds that a beneficiary's questionnaire fails to note the existence of other health plan coverage.

Providers and suppliers are required to complete information on claim forms regarding potential coverage under other plans. Civil monetary penalties are established for an entity that knowingly, willfully, and repeatedly fails to complete a claim form with accurate information.

Contractors are required to submit annually a report to the Centers for Medicare & Medicaid Services regarding steps taken to recover mistaken payments.

B-5. Can a person age 65 or over qualify for Hospital Insurance (Part A) benefits without qualifying for Social Security or Railroad Retirement benefits?

Most persons age 65 or over and otherwise ineligible for Hospital Insurance may enroll voluntarily and pay a monthly premium if they are also enrolled for Medical Insurance. (See C-1.)

Most persons who reached age 65 before 1968 are eligible to enroll for Hospital Insurance for which no premiums need to be paid even if they have no coverage under Social Security. Also eligible for enrollment under this transitional provision are persons age 65 and over with specified amounts of earnings credits less than that required for cash benefit eligibility.

Not eligible under the transitional provision are (1) retired federal employees covered by the Federal Employees' Health Benefits Act of 1959, (2) non-residents of the United States, and (3) aliens admitted for permanent residence (unless lawfully admitted for permanent residence in the United States continuously during the five years immediately preceding the month in which they apply for enrollment).

B-6. Is there any way that an individual not eligible for Hospital Insurance (Part A) can be enrolled?

Yes, provided the individual (1) has attained age 65, (2) is enrolled in Medical Insurance (see SECTION C), (3) is a resident of the United States and is either (a) a citizen, or (b) an alien lawfully admitted for permanent residence who has resided in the United States continuously during the five years immediately preceding the month in which he applies for enrollment, and (4) is not otherwise entitled to Hospital Insurance benefits.

Disabled individuals under age 65 may also be able to obtain Hospital Insurance coverage through monthly premiums. The Omnibus Budget Reconciliation Act of 1989 extended eligibility to individuals under age 65 who qualify for Hospital Insurance benefits on the basis of a disabling physical or mental impairment, but who lose entitlement because they have earnings that exceed the eligibility limit for Social Security disability benefits and are not otherwise entitled to Hospital Insurance benefits.

The Hospital Insurance premium is $410 a month in 2007 (but see paragraph below for premium reduction exception). This premium amount increases by 10% for those who must pay a premium surcharge for late enrollment. (See C-2 and C-3.)

The Hospital Insurance premium is reduced, on a phased-in basis, for individuals and their spouses with credits for 30 or more quarters paid into the Social Security system. The Hospital Insurance premium is reduced by approximately 45% (to $226 a month in 2007). The reduction in premium payments will also apply to the surviving spouse or divorced spouse of an individual who had at least 30 quarters of coverage under Social Security. This premium amount increases by 10% for those who must pay a premium surcharge of late enrollment. (See C-2 and C-3.)

An individual who qualifies for the reduction is an individual who (1) has 30 or more quarters of coverage, (2) has been married for at least the previous one year period to a worker who has 30 or more quarters of coverage, (3) had been married to a worker who had 30 or more quarters of coverage for a period of at least one year before the death of the worker, (4) is divorced from, after at least 10 years of marriage to, a worker who had 30 or more quarters of coverage at the time the divorce became final, or (5) is divorced from, after at least 10 years of marriage to, a worker who subsequently died and who had 30 or more quarters of coverage at the time the divorce became final.

Beginning January 1, 1998, certain public employment retirees are no longer required to pay a premium to receive Hospital Insurance benefits. Such individuals include those (1) receiving cash benefits under qualified state or local government retirement systems generally, or on the basis of employment for at least 40 calendar quarters, (2) married for at least one year to someone with at least 40 quarters of coverage, (3) that had been married for at least one year to a person with at least 40 quarters of coverage before death, (4) that are divorced from a person (after at least 10 years of marriage) with at least 40 quarters of coverage, or (5) those whose Hospital Insurance premium will not be paid (or had not been paid for the prior 84 months) by a state (including Medicaid).

ADMINISTRATION

B-7. How does the Centers for Medicare & Medicaid Services administer Hospital Insurance (Part A)?

The Centers for Medicare & Medicaid Services enters into agreements with state agencies and with fiscal intermediaries (such as Blue Cross and other health insurance organizations) to administer Hospital Insurance.

State agencies survey institutions to determine whether they meet the conditions for participation as a hospital, skilled nursing facility, home health agency, or hospice. They also help the institutions meet the conditions for participation.

Private organizations called fiscal intermediaries determine the amount of Hospital Insurance benefits payable to hospitals, skilled nursing facilities, hospices, and home health agencies; pay hospital insurance benefits to hospitals, skilled nursing facilities, hospices, and home health agencies out of funds advanced by the federal government; help hospitals, skilled nursing facilities, hospices, and home health agencies establish and maintain necessary financial records; serve as a channel of communication of information relating to the Hospital Insurance protection; and audit records of hospitals, skilled nursing facilities, hospices, and home health agencies, as necessary, to insure that payment of Hospital Insurance benefits is proper.

Each provider of services can nominate a fiscal intermediary to work with or can deal directly with the Centers for Medicare & Medicaid Services. Fiscal intermediaries are reimbursed for their reasonable costs of administration.

Most skilled nursing facilities and home health agencies must submit cost reports to fiscal intermediaries in a standardized electronic format. Hospitals have been required to submit cost reports in electronic format for a number of years. No payments are made to a provider unless it has furnished the information needed to determine the amount of payments due the provider. In general, providers submit this information through cost reports that cover a 12-month period. A provider may request a delay or waiver of the electronic submission requirement by submitting a written request with supporting documentation to its fiscal intermediary no later than 30 days after the end of its cost reporting period.

B-8. What is the Prospective Payment System?

Medicare pays for most inpatient hospital care under the Prospective Payment System (PPS). Under PPS, hospitals are paid a predetermined rate per discharge for inpatient services furnished to Medicare beneficiaries. The predetermined rates are based on payment categories called Diagnosis Related Groups, or DRGs. In some cases, Medicare payment will be more than the hospital's cost; in other cases, the payment will be less than the hospital's costs. In special cases, where costs for necessary care are unusually high or the length of stay is unusually long, the hospital receives additional payment.

Reimbursement for inpatient hospital services is based on uniform sums for about 475 DRGs (varying between rural and urban facilities). All other services are reimbursed on a reasonable cost basis.

Health Maintenance Organizations (HMOs) are covered by special reimbursement provisions to reward them financially because of what is believed to be their more favorable operating experience.

The PPS system does not change Hospital Insurance protection. PPS does not determine the length of a stay in the hospital or the extent of care a patient receives, but is a factor providers consider when providing covered care. The law requires participating hospitals to accept Medicare payments as payment in full, and those hospitals are prohibited from billing the Medicare patient for anything other than the applicable deductible and coinsurance amounts, plus any amounts due for noncovered items or services such as television, telephone or private duty nurses. This must be done even when the cost of the patient's care greatly exceeds the payment the hospital will receive from Medicare.

Despite the requirement to provide care for as long as it is medically necessary, the PPS provides hospitals with the possible incentive to refuse to admit patients for medical procedures that might not be reimbursed by Medicare. Hospitals also have the incentive to treat and discharge patients within or less than the time frame established by the reimbursement rate for a particular DRG.

The Centers for Medicare & Medicaid Services contracts with quality improvement organizations (QIOs) in each state to conduct preadmission, continued stay, and retrospective reviews of the services delivered by a hospital. The reviews determine whether such services are reasonable and necessary. The QIO is also responsible for ensuring that the cost control incentives of the PPS do not adversely affect patients' access to hospitals or the quality of hospital care.

If the hospital, without consulting the QIO, recommends against admitting a patient, review of this decision may be obtained by the patient by writing the QIO in the patient's state. If the QIO participated in the preadmission denial of the patient, then a reconsideration of that denial may be requested by the patient.

For a detailed explanation of the appeal process, see SECTION F.

B-9. Is Hospital Insurance (Part A) a compulsory program?

Yes. Every person who works in employment or self-employment covered by the Social Security Act, or in employment covered by the Railroad Retirement Act, must pay the Hospital Insurance tax. They will be eligible for Hospital Insurance benefits if fully insured when they reach age 65, receive disability benefits for more than 24 months, or have end-stage renal disease.

FINANCING HOSPITAL INSURANCE (PART A)

B-10. How is Hospital Insurance (Part A) financed?

By a separate Hospital Insurance tax imposed upon employers, employees, and the self-employed. The tax must be paid by every individual, regardless of age, who is subject to the regular Social Security tax or to the Railroad Retirement tax. It must also be paid by all federal employees and by all state and local government employees (1) hired after

March 1986, or (2) not covered by a state retirement system in conjunction with their employment (beginning July 2, 1991). The tax is imposed upon all earnings. The rates of the Hospital Insurance tax are 1.45% each for employees and employers, and 2.90% for self-employed persons.

There is a special federal (and generally following through to state) income tax deduction of 50% of the OASDI/Hospital Insurance self-employment tax. This income tax deduction, which is available regardless of whether or not the taxpayer itemizes deductions, is designed to treat the self-employed in much the same manner as employees and employers are treated for Social Security and income tax purposes.

BENEFITS

B-11. In general, what benefits are provided under Hospital Insurance?

Over and above the "deductible" and "coinsurance" amounts which must be paid by the patient, the following services are covered:

(1) *Inpatient hospital care* for up to 90 days in each "benefit period." The patient pays a deductible of $992 in 2007 for the first 60 days and coinsurance of $248 a day for each additional day up to a maximum of 30 days. In addition, each person has a non-renewable lifetime "reserve" of 60 additional hospital days with coinsurance of $496 a day.

(2) *Posthospital extended care in a skilled nursing facility* for up to 100 days in each "benefit period." The patient pays nothing for the first 20 days in 2007. After 20 days the patient pays coinsurance of $124.00 a day for each additional day up to a maximum of 80 days.

(3) The first 100 *post-hospital home health service* visits following a hospital or skilled nursing facility stay. The services must be made under a plan of treatment established by a physician, except that there is 20% cost-sharing payable by the patient for durable medical equipment (other than the purchase of certain used items).

(4) *Hospice care* for terminally ill patients.

QUALIFIED MEDICARE BENEFICIARIES

B-12. When will a state pay Medicare costs for a person who is elderly or disabled with low income?

Federal law requires state Medicaid programs to pay Medicare costs for certain elderly and disabled persons with low incomes and very limited resources.

There are two programs to help people pay their Medicare expenses. One is called the "Qualified Medicare Beneficiary" or "QMB" program. The other is called the "Specified Low-Income Medicare Beneficiary" or "SLMB" program.

The QMB program is for persons with limited resources whose incomes are at or below the national poverty level. It covers the cost of Medicare premiums, coinsurance, and deductibles that Medicare beneficiaries normally pay out of their own pockets. If a person qualifies for assistance under the QMB program, he will not have to pay:

- Medicare's hospital deductible ($992 per benefit period in 2007).

- The daily coinsurance charges for extended hospital and skilled nursing facility stays.

- The Medicare Medical Insurance (Part B) premium, which is $93.50 per month (for most individuals) in 2007.

- The annual Part B deductible of $131 for 2007.

- The 20% coinsurance for services covered by Medicare Part B, depending on which doctor the patient goes to.

The state covers these Medicare cost sharing amounts. The patient is only responsible for paying for the various medical supplies and services not covered by Medicare, such as routine physicals, dental care, hearing aids, and eyeglasses.

While the QMB programs helps those whose income is at or below the national poverty level, the SLMB program is for persons whose incomes are slightly higher than the poverty level, but not more than 20% higher. If a person qualifies for assistance under the SLMB program, the state will pay the monthly Part B premium. The patient will, however, continue to be responsible for Medicare's deductibles, coinsurance, and for charges for health care services and medical supplies not covered by Medicare.

B-13. How does a person qualify for assistance under the QMB program?

The rules may vary from state to state but, in general terms, to qualify for assistance under the QMB program, a person must meet the following requirements:

(1) The person must be entitled to Hospital Insurance (Part A). If the person does not have Part A or does not know whether he is entitled to Part A, check with any Social Security Administration office or call 1-800-772-1213.

(2) The person's financial resources, such as bank accounts, stocks, and bonds, cannot exceed $4,000 for one person or $6,000 for a couple. Some things–the home you live in, one automobile, burial plots, home furnishings, personal jewelry, and life insurance–usually do not count as resources.

(3) The person's income must be at or below the national poverty level. The QMB annual income limits in 2007 until adjusted not later than April 1, 2007 are $9,804 for an individual, and $13,200 for a couple. The income limits are higher in Alaska and Hawaii. Income includes, but is not limited to, Social Security benefits, pensions, and wages. Interest payments and dividends can also count as income.

B-14. What if a person's income is slightly higher than the poverty level?

If a person does not qualify for QMB assistance because his income is too high, he may be able to get help under the Specified Low-Income Beneficiary (SLMB) program. To qualify for SLMB assistance, a person must meet the following requirements:

(1) The person must be entitled to Hospital Insurance (Part A). If the person does not have Part A or does not know whether he is entitled to Part A, check with any Social Security Administration office or call 1-800-772-1213.

(2) A person's financial resources, such as bank accounts, stocks, and bonds, cannot exceed $4,000 for one person or $6,000 for a couple. The following usually do not count as resources: the home you live in, one automobile, burial plots, home furnishings, personal jewelry, and life insurance.

(3) A person's income cannot exceed the national poverty level by more than 20%. This means that in 2006, and until adjusted, not later than April 1, 2007, the SLMB income limits are $11,760 annually for an individual, and $15,840 annually for a couple.

B-15. How does a person apply for QMB or SLMB assistance?

A person with Hospital Insurance (Part A) must file an application for Medicare assistance programs at a state, county, or local medical assistance office. A person without Hospital Insurance (Part A) should contact a Social Security Administration office.

INPATIENT HOSPITAL SERVICES

B-16. Specifically, what inpatient hospital services are paid for under Hospital Insurance?

Except for the "deductible" and "coinsurance" amounts that must be paid by the patient, Medicare helps pay for inpatient hospital service for up to 90 days in each "benefit period." Medicare will also pay (except for a coinsurance amount) for 60 additional hospital days over each person's lifetime (applies to disabled beneficiaries at any age; others after age 65).

Medicare pays for hospital care if the patient meets the following four conditions: (1) a doctor prescribes inpatient hospital care for treatment of the illness or injury, (2) the patient requires the kind of care that can only be provided in a hospital, (3) the hospital is participating in Medicare, and (4) the Utilization Review Committee of the hospital, a Quality Improvement Organization (QIO), or an intermediary does not disapprove of the stay.

The patient must pay a "deductible" of $992 in 2007 for the first 60 days in each benefit period. If the stay is longer than 60 days during a benefit period, "coinsurance" of $248 a day must be paid for each additional day up to a maximum of 30 days.

Thus, a 90-day stay would cost the patient $8,432. After 90 days, the patient pays the full bill unless the lifetime reserve of 60 days is drawn upon. The patient must pay coinsurance of $496 a day for these 60 additional "lifetime reserve" days.

The coinsurance amounts are based on those in effect when services are furnished, rather than on those in effect at the beginning of the beneficiary's spell of illness (benefit period).

The 90-day benefit period starts again with each spell of illness. A "benefit period" is a way of measuring the patient's use of services under Hospital Insurance. The patient's first benefit period starts the first time the patient receives inpatient hospital care after Hospital Insurance begins. A benefit period ends when the patient has been out of a hospital or other facility primarily providing skilled nursing or rehabilitative services for 60 days in a row (including the day of discharge). If a patient remains in a facility (other than a hospital) that primarily provides skilled nursing or rehabilitative services, a benefit period ends when the patient has not received any skilled care there for 60 days in a row. After one benefit period has ended, another one will start whenever the patient again receives inpatient hospital care.

There is no limit to the number of 90-day benefit periods a person can have in a lifetime (except in the case of hospitalization for mental illness). But the "lifetime reserve" of 60 days is not renewable. Also, special limited benefit periods apply to hospice care. (See B-24.)

Example. Mr. Smith enters the hospital on February 5. He is discharged on February 15. He has used 10 days of his first benefit period. Mr. Smith is not hospitalized again until August 20. Since more than 60 days elapsed between his hospital stays, he begins a new benefit period, his Hospital Insurance coverage is completely renewed, and he will again pay the hospital deductible.

Example. Mr. Jones enters the hospital on September 14. He is discharged on September 24. He also has used 10 days of his first benefit period. But he is then readmitted to the hospital on October 20. Since fewer than 60 days elapsed between hospital stays, Mr. Jones is still in his first benefit period and will not be required to pay another hospital deductible. This means that the first day of his second admission is counted as the eleventh day of hospital care in that benefit period. Mr. Jones will not begin a new benefit period until he has been out of the hospital (and has not received any skilled care in a skilled nursing facility) for 60 consecutive days.

"Lifetime reserve" days include an extra 60 hospital days a patient can use if the patient has a long illness and needs to stay in the hospital for more than 90 days. A patient has only 60 reserve days in a lifetime. For example, if a patient uses 8 reserve days in his first hospital stay this year, the next time he visits a hospital he will have only 52 reserve days left to use, whether or not he has a new benefit period. A patient can decide when he wants to use his reserve days. After a patient has been in the hospital 90 days, the patient can use all or some of his 60 reserve days if he wishes.

If a patient does not want to use his reserve days, the patient must tell the hospital in writing, either when he is admitted to the hospital, or at any time afterwards up to 90 days after he has been discharged. If a patient uses reserve days and then decides that he did not want to use them, the patient must request approval from the hospital to have them restored. During 2007, Hospital Insurance (Part A) pays for all covered services except $496 a day for each reserve day the patient uses.

Medicare beneficiaries have the right to receive all the hospital care that is necessary for the proper diagnosis and treatment of their illness or injury. Under federal law, a beneficiary's discharge date must be determined solely by medical needs, not by the diagnosis related group (DRG) or Medicare payments. Beneficiaries have the right to be fully informed about decisions affecting their Medicare coverage and payment for their hospital stay and for any post-hospital services. They also have the right to request a review by a quality improvement organization (QIO) of any written notice of noncoverage they receive from the hospital stating that Medicare will no longer pay for their hospital care. QIOs are groups of doctors who are paid by the federal government to review medical necessity, appropriateness and quality of hospital treatment furnished to Medicare patients. (See B-8.)

The following inpatient services are covered by Hospital Insurance (Part A):

- *Bed and board in a semi-private room* (two to four beds) or a ward (five or more beds). Hospital Insurance will pay the cost of a private room only if it is required for medical reasons (e.g., the patient needs isolation for medical reasons or needs immediate hospitalization and no other accommodations are available). If the patient requests a private room, Hospital Insurance will pay the cost of semi-private accommodations; the patient must pay the extra charge for the private room. The patient or family must be told the amount of this extra charge when a private room is requested. Normally, Medicare patients are assigned to semi-private rooms. Ward assignments are made only under extraordinary circumstances.

- *All meals*, including special diets.

- *Nursing services* provided by or under the supervision of licensed nursing personnel (other than the services of a private duty nurse or attendant).

- Services of the hospital's *medical social workers*.

- Use of regular hospital *equipment, supplies, and appliances*, such as oxygen tents, wheel chairs, crutches, casts, surgical dressings, splints, and hospital "admission packs" (toilet articles) when routinely furnished by the hospital to all patients. Certain equipment, supplies and appliances used by the patient in the hospital continue to be covered after the patient has been discharged. Examples include a cardiac pacemaker and an artificial limb.

- *Drugs and biologicals* ordinarily furnished by the hospital. A limited supply of drugs needed for use outside the hospital is also covered, but only if medically necessary in order to facilitate the patient's departure from the hospital and the supply is necessary until the patient can obtain a continuing supply. Drugs and biologicals that the hospital obtains for the patient from a private source (community pharmacy) are covered when the hospital is responsible for making payment to the supplier.

- *Diagnostic or therapeutic items and services* ordinarily furnished by the hospital or by others (including clinical psychologists, as defined by the Centers for Medicare & Medicaid Services), under arrangements made with the hospital.

- *Operating and recovery room costs*, including hospital costs for anesthesia services.

- Services of *interns and residents in training* under an approved teaching program.

- *Blood transfusions*, after the first three pints. Hospital Insurance helps pay for blood (whole blood or units of packed red blood cells), blood components, and the cost of blood processing and administration. If the patient receives blood as an inpatient of a hospital or skilled nursing facility, Hospital Insurance will pay for these blood costs, except for any nonreplacement fees charged for the first three pints of whole blood or units of packed red cells per calendar year. The nonreplacement fee is the amount that some hospitals and skilled nursing facilities charge for blood that is not replaced. The patient is responsible for the nonreplacement fees for the first three pints or units of blood furnished by a hospital or skilled nursing facility. If the patient is charged nonreplacement fees, the patient has the option of either paying the fees or having the blood replaced. If the patient chooses to have the blood replaced, the patient can either replace the blood personally or arrange to have another person or an organization replace it. A hospital or skilled nursing facility cannot charge a patient for any of the first three pints of blood that the patient replaces or arranges to replace. If the patient has already paid for or replaced blood under Medical Insurance (Part B) of Medicare during the calendar year, the patient does not have to meet those costs again under Hospital Insurance.

- *X-rays* and other radiology services, including radiation therapy, billed by the hospital.

- *Lab tests*.

- *Respiratory or inhalation therapy*.

- *Independent clinical laboratory services* under arrangement with the hospital.

- *Alcohol detoxification and rehabilitation services* when furnished as inpatient hospital services. Alcohol detoxification and rehabilitation services are also covered under Medical Insurance (Part B) when furnished as physician services.

- *Dental services* when the patient requires hospitalization because of the severity of the dental procedure or because of his underlying medical condition and clinical status.

- Cost of *special care units*, such as an intensive care unit, coronary care unit, etc.

- *Rehabilitation services*, such as physical therapy, occupational therapy, and speech pathology services.

- *Appliances* (such as pacemakers, colostomy fittings, and artificial limbs) which are permanently installed while in the hospital.

- *Lung and heart-lung transplants.* (See C-40 for additional information on this coverage and what benefits are covered under Hospital Insurance (Part A) or Medical Insurance (Part B.))

Hospital Insurance does *not* pay for

- Services of physicians and surgeons, including the services of pathologists, radiologists, anesthesiologists, and physiatrists. (Nor does Hospital Insurance pay for the services of a physician, resident physician or intern–except those provided by an intern or resident in training under an approved teaching program.)

- Services of a private duty nurse or attendant, unless the patient's condition requires such services and the nurse or attendant is a bona fide employee of the hospital.

- Personal convenience items supplied at the patient's request, such as television rental, radio rental, or telephone.

- The first three pints of whole blood (or packed red blood cells) received in a calendar year.

- Supplies, appliances and equipment for use outside the hospital, unless continued use is required (e.g., a pacemaker).

B-17. Are inpatient hospital benefits provided for care in a psychiatric hospital?

Yes, but benefits for psychiatric hospital care are subject to a lifetime limit of 190 days. Furthermore, if the patient is already in a mental hospital when he becomes eligible for Medicare, the time spent there in the 150-day period before becoming eligible will be counted against the maximum of 150 days available in such cases (including any later period of such hospitalization when he has not been out of a mental hospital for at least 60 consecutive days between hospitalizations). However, this latter limitation does not apply to inpatient service in a general hospital for other than psychiatric care.

B-18. What special provisions apply to care in religious nonmedical health care institutions?

In general, these institutions can participate in Medicare as hospitals, and the regular coverages and exclusions relating to inpatient hospital care will apply. Thus, the patient pays a $992 deductible in 2007 for the first 60 days, and coinsurance of $248 a day in 2007 for the next 30 days (plus $496 a day in 2007 for the 60 lifetime reserve days). A religious nonmedical health care institution may also be paid as a skilled nursing facility. But extended care benefits will be paid for only 30 days in a calendar year (instead of the usual 100 days), and the patient must pay the coinsurance amount ($124.00 a day in 2007) for each day of service (instead of only for each day after the 20th day).

A federal district court ruled in 1996 that certain Christian Science facilities were not eligible for Medicare and Medicaid payments. In response to the ruling, Congress deleted any references to Christian Science sanatoriums in the Social Security Act and replaced them with the term "religious nonmedical health care institutions." The Balanced Budget Act of 1997 includes detailed eligibility criteria for facilities to protect the health and safety of patients, and limits the total amount of expenditures that can be paid to religious nonmedical health care institutions.

B-19. Can patients choose their own hospitals?

Except for certain emergency cases, Medicare will make payments to "qualified" hospitals, skilled nursing facilities, home health agencies, and hospices only.

Medicare generally does not pay for hospital or medical services outside the United States. (Puerto Rico, the U.S. Virgin Islands, Guam, American Samoa, and the Northern Mariana Islands are considered part of the United States.)

There are rare emergency cases where Medicare will pay for care in Canada or Mexico. Also, Medicare will sometimes pay a Mexican or Canadian hospital if it is closer to the home of a United States resident than the nearest United States hospital. But such hospitals must be approved. Medicare also authorizes payment for emergency care in a Canadian hospital when the emergency occurred in the United States or in transit between Alaska and other continental states. Necessary physicians' services in connection with Mexican or Canadian hospitalization are authorized under Medicare's Medical Insurance. If a person receives emergency treatment in a Canadian or Mexican hospital or lives near a Canadian or Mexican hospital, he should have the hospital help him contact a Medicare intermediary.

B-20. Must a doctor certify that hospitalization is required?

Initial certification is no longer required except for inpatient psychiatric hospital services and inpatient tuberculosis hospital services. For prolonged hospital stays, however, certification by a doctor may be required.

B-21. What must a hospital or Health Maintenance Organization do to qualify for Medicare payments?

The hospital must meet certain standards and enter into a Medicare agreement. However, Medicare may pay nonparticipating hospitals where emergency care is given.

HOSPICE CARE

B-22. What is hospice care?

Hospice care is an approach to treatment that recognizes that the impending death of an individual warrants a change in focus from curative care to palliative care (relief of pain and other uncomfortable symptoms). The goal of hospice care is to help terminally ill individuals continue life with minimal disruption to normal activities while remaining primarily in the home environment. A hospice uses an interdisciplinary approach to deliver medical, social, psychological, emotional, and spiritual services through the use of a broad spectrum of professional and other caregivers, with the goal of making the individual as physically and emotionally comfortable as possible. Counseling and respite services are available to the family of the hospice patient. Hospice programs consider both the patient and the family as a unit of care.

The Social Security Act provides coverage for hospice care for terminally ill Medicare beneficiaries who elect to receive care from a participating hospice.

A hospice is a public agency or private organization that is primarily engaged in providing pain relief, symptom management, and supportive services to terminally ill people.

B-23. How is hospice care covered under Medicare?

Under the Medicare hospice benefit, Medicare pays for services every day and also permits a hospice to provide appropriate custodial care, including homemaker services and counseling. Hospice care under Medicare includes both home care and inpatient care, when needed, and a variety of services not otherwise covered under Medicare.

Medicare payments to a hospice are based on one of four prospectively determined rates for each day in which a qualified Medicare beneficiary is under the care of the hospice. The four rate categories are routine home care, continuous home care, inpatient respite care, and general inpatient care. Payment rates are adjusted to reflect local differences in area wage levels.

Hospice care is covered under Hospital Insurance (Part A) when the beneficiary (1) is eligible for Hospital Insurance benefits, (2) is certified by a doctor as terminally ill (i.e., life expectancy of six months or less), and (3) files a statement electing to waive all other Medicare coverage for hospice care from hospice programs other than the one chosen, and elects not to receive other services related to treatment of the terminal condition. (The beneficiary can later revoke the election.)

The following are covered hospice services:

- Nursing care provided by or under the supervision of a registered professional nurse.

- Medical social services provided by a social worker under a physician's direction.

- Counseling (including dietary counseling) with respect to care of the terminally ill patient and adjustment to his approaching death.

- Short-term inpatient care (including both respite care and procedures necessary for pain control and acute and chronic symptom management) provided in a participating hospice, hospital, or skilled nursing facility. The respite care may be provided only on an intermittent, nonroutine, and occasional basis and may not be provided consecutively over longer than five days.

- Medical appliances and supplies.

- Services of a home health aide and homemaker services.

- Drugs, including outpatient drugs for pain relief and symptom management.

- Physical therapy, occupational therapy, and speech-language pathology services to control symptoms or to enable the patient to maintain activities of daily living and basic functional skills.

Services of a home health aide, homemaker services, and nursing care provided by or under the supervision of a registered professional nurse, may be provided on a 24-hour, continuous basis only during periods of crisis and only as necessary to maintain the terminally ill patient at home.

The definition of hospice care also includes any other item or service which is specified in the patient's plan of care and for which Medicare may pay.

According to the *Social Security Act*, a "hospice program" is a public agency or private organization which is primarily engaged in providing the care and services listed above and makes the services available (as needed) on a 24-hour basis. A hospice program also provides bereavement counseling for the immediate family of the terminally ill patient. The care and services must be provided in the patient's home, on an outpatient basis, and on a short-term inpatient basis. The nursing, physician, counseling, and medical social service benefits must be provided directly on a routine basis. The remaining hospice benefits may be provided through arrangements with other hospice programs (provided the agency or organization maintains professional management responsibility for all services).

The Centers for Medicare & Medicaid Services may waive certain service requirements for hospices not located in urbanized areas that can demonstrate that they have been unable, despite diligent efforts, to recruit appropriate personnel. For these hospices, the Centers for Medicare & Medicaid Services may waive the provision requiring physical or occupational therapy or speech-language pathology services and dietary counseling.

A hospice program must have an interdisciplinary group of personnel (at least one physician, one registered nurse, one social worker, and one pastoral or other counselor) to establish the policies of the program and provide the required care and services. The group must maintain central clinical records on all patients, utilize volunteers, and is required to continue hospice care for any patient who is unable to pay for such care.

B-24. What is the hospice benefit period?

The benefit period consists of two 90-day periods followed by an unlimited number of 60-day periods. The medical director or physician member of the hospice interdisciplinary team must re-certify that the beneficiary is terminally ill at the beginning of the 60-day periods.

B-25. What does the patient pay for hospice care?

There are no deductibles under the hospice benefit. The beneficiary does not pay for Medicare-covered services for the terminal illness, except for small coinsurance amounts for outpatient drugs and inpatient respite care. For outpatient prescription drugs, the patient is responsible for 5% of the cost of drugs or $5, whichever is less. For inpatient respite care, the patient pays 5% of the amount paid by Medicare for a respite care day.

The amount paid by Medicare is equal to the reasonable costs of providing hospice care or based on other tests of reasonableness as prescribed by regulations. No payment may be made for bereavement counseling, and no reimbursement may be made for other counseling services (including nutritional and dietary counseling) as separate services.

B-26. How is respite care covered?

Respite care as an inpatient in a hospice (to give a period of relief to the family providing home care for the patient) is limited to no more than five days in a row. Respite care requires coinsurance in the amount of 5% of the amount that Medicare pays for the respite care. This coinsurance amount may not exceed the inpatient hospital deductible.

SKILLED NURSING FACILITY CARE

B-27. What is a qualified skilled nursing facility?

A skilled nursing facility is a specially qualified facility that specializes in skilled care. It has the staff and equipment to provide skilled nursing care or skilled rehabilitative services and other related health services.

A skilled nursing facility may be a skilled nursing home, or a distinct part of an institution, such as a ward or wing of a hospital, or a section of a facility another part of which is an old-age home. Not all nursing homes will qualify; those which offer only custodial care are excluded. The facility must be primarily engaged in providing skilled nursing care or rehabilitation services for injured, disabled or sick persons. Skilled nursing care means care that can only be performed by, or under the supervision of, licensed nursing personnel. Skilled rehabilitation services may include such services as physical therapy performed by, or under the supervision of, a professional therapist.

At least one registered nurse must be employed full-time and adequate nursing service (which may include practical nurses) must be provided at all times. Every patient must be under the supervision of a doctor, and a doctor must always be available for emergency care. Generally, the facility must be certified by the state. It also must have a written agreement with a hospital that is participating in the Medicare program for the transfer of patients.

Skilled nursing care is care that can only be performed by, or under the supervision of, licensed nursing personnel. Skilled nursing care and skilled rehabilitation services must be needed and received on a daily basis (at least five days a week) or the patient is not eligible for Medicare coverage.

A skilled nursing facility must provide 24-hour nursing service and must employ a registered professional nurse during a day tour of duty of at least 8 hours a day, seven days a week. The facility must require that the medical care of every resident be provided under the supervision of a physician, and have a physician available to furnish necessary medical care in case of emergency.

Many residents of nursing homes will not qualify for Medicare coverage because coverage is restricted to patients in need of skilled nursing and rehabilitative services on a daily basis.

The initial determination of Medicare coverage is made by the nursing home, but the nursing home cannot charge the patient for care provided before it notifies the patient in writing that it believes Medicare will not pay for the care. The patient may not challenge the nursing home's non-coverage determination until a claim has been submitted to and denied by the Medicare intermediary. The patient does have the right to require a nursing home to submit its claim to the Medicare intermediary so that the intermediary can determine if the nursing home was correct in denying coverage.

Skilled nursing facilities must provide patients with the following rights: (1) equal access and admission, (2) notice of rights and services, (3) transfer and discharge rights, (4) the right to pretransfer and predischarge notice, (5) access and visitation rights, (6) rights relating to the protection of resident funds, and (7) certain other specified rights.

An institution which is primarily for the care and treatment of mental diseases or tuberculosis is not a skilled nursing facility.

Most nursing homes in the United States are *not* skilled nursing facilities and many skilled nursing facilities are not certified by Medicare. In some facilities, only certain portions participate in Medicare. Medicare does not pay for custodial care when that is the only kind of care needed. Care is considered custodial when it is primarily for the purpose of helping the patient with daily living or meeting personal needs, and could be provided safely and reasonably by people without professional skills or training. For example, custodial care includes help in walking, getting in and out of bed, bathing, dressing, eating, and taking medicine.

B-28. What provisions are made under Hospital Insurance for care in a skilled nursing facility or other such facility?

In order to qualify for skilled nursing facility benefits under Hospital Insurance, the patient must meet all of these five conditions:

(1) The patient's condition requires daily skilled nursing or skilled rehabilitative services which, as a practical matter, can only be provided in a skilled nursing facility.

(2) The patient has been in a hospital at least three days in a row (not counting the day of discharge) before being admitted to a participating skilled nursing facility.

(3) The patient is admitted to the skilled nursing facility within a short time (generally within 30 days) after leaving the hospital.

(4) The patient's care in the skilled nursing facility is for a condition that was treated in the hospital, or for a condition that arose while receiving care in the skilled nursing facility for a condition which was treated in the hospital.

(5) A medical professional certifies that the patient needs, and receives, skilled nursing or skilled rehabilitation services (post-hospital extended care) on a daily basis.

Exception. Skilled nursing facility coverage is permitted without regard to the three-day prior hospital stay requirement if there is no increase in cost to the program involved, and the acute care nature of the benefit is not altered. Persons covered without a prior hospital stay may be subject to limitations in the scope of or extent of services. The Department of Health and Human Services will decide when to lift the three-day prior hospital stay requirement but has not done so yet (and is not likely to do so).

If a patient leaves a skilled nursing facility and is readmitted within 30 days, the patient does not need to have a new three-day stay in a hospital for care to be covered.

Doctor's services are not covered by Hospital Insurance when the patient is in a skilled nursing facility. Medicare Medical Insurance (Part B) covers doctor's services.

Except for a coinsurance amount payable by the patient after the first 20 days, Hospital Insurance (Part A) will pay the reasonable cost of post-hospital care in a skilled nursing facility for up to 100 days in a benefit period.

The following items and services are covered:

- Bed and board in a semi-private room (two to four beds in a room), unless the patient's condition requires isolation or no semi-private rooms are available.

- Nursing care provided by, or under the supervision of, a registered nurse (but not private-duty nursing).

- Drugs, biologicals, supplies (such as splints and casts), appliances (such as wheelchairs) and equipment for use in the facility.

- Medical social services. According to the *Medicare Intermediary Manual*, these services can include a wide assortment of services, including the assessment of the patient's medical and nursing requirements, and the patient's financial resources, home situation, and the community services available to him. They can also include the assessment of the social and emotional factors related to the patient's illness, and the patient's need for care, response to treatment, and adjustment to care in the skilled nursing facility. Appropriate action to obtain case work services to assist in resolving problems in these areas is covered by Medicare.

- Medical services of interns and residents in training under an approved teaching program of a hospital.

- Other diagnostic or therapeutic services provided by a hospital with which the facility has a transfer agreement.

- Rehabilitation services, such as physical, occupational, and speech therapy, furnished by the skilled nursing facility, or by others under arrangements made by the skilled nursing facility.

- All meals, including special diets furnished by the facility.

- Blood transfusions, other than the first three pints of blood.

- Such other health services as are generally provided by a skilled nursing facility.

The following services are *not* covered:

- Personal convenience items that the patient requests, such as a television, radio, or telephone.

- Private duty nurses or attendants.

- Any extra charges for a private room, unless it is determined to be medically necessary.

- Custodial care, including assistance with the activities of daily living (i.e., walking, getting in and out of bed, bathing, dressing, and feeding), special diets, and supervision of medication that can usually be self-administered.

Federal regulations include the following services for skilled rehabilitation and nursing care: (1) insertion and sterile irrigation and replacement of catheters, (2) application of dressing involving prescription medications and aseptic techniques, (3) treatment of extensive bed sores or other widespread skin disorders, (4) therapeutic exercises or activities supervised or performed by a qualified occupational or physical therapist, (5) training to restore a patient's ability to walk, and (6) range of motion exercises that are part of a physical therapist's active treatment to restore a patient's mobility.

A number of services involving the development, management and evaluation of a patient care plan may qualify as skilled services. These services are "skilled" if the patient's condition requires the services to be provided or supervised by a professional to meet the patient's needs, promote recovery, and ensure the patient's medical safety. For example, a patient with a history of diabetes and heart problems, who is recovering from a broken arm, may require skin care, medication, a special diet, an exercise program to preserve muscle tone, and observation to detect signs of deterioration or complications. Although none of these required services are "skilled" on their own, the combination, provided by a professional, may be considered "skilled."

To qualify for skilled nursing facility reimbursement, skilled physical therapy must be (1) specifically related to a physician's active treatment plan, (2) of a complexity, or involve a condition, that requires a physical therapist, (3) necessary to establish a safe maintenance program or provided where the patient's condition will improve within a predictable time, and (4) of the necessary frequency and duration.

B-29. How much does the patient pay for skilled nursing facility care?

The patient pays nothing for the first 20 days of covered services in each spell of illness; after 20 days, coinsurance is payable for each additional day, up to a maximum of 80 days. For a patient in a skilled nursing facility in 2007, the coinsurance is $124.00 a day.

Thus, a 100-day stay in a skilled nursing facility during 2007 will cost the patient $9,920.

There is no lifetime limit on the amount of skilled nursing facility care provided under Hospital Insurance. Except for the coinsurance (which must be paid after the first 20 days in each spell of illness), the plan will pay the cost of 100 days' post-hospital care in each benefit period, regardless of how many benefit periods the person may have. After 100 days of coverage, the patient must pay the full cost of skilled nursing facility care.

Skilled nursing facilities cannot require a patient to pay a deposit or other payment as a condition of admission to the facility unless it is clear that services are not covered under Medicare.

B-30. When can payment be made for skilled nursing care?

Payment will be made for skilled nursing care only if the following conditions are met:

(1) The beneficiary files a written request for payment (another person may sign the request if it is impracticable for the patient to sign).

(2) A physician certifies that the patient needs skilled nursing care on an inpatient basis. Recertification is required for extended stays.

(3) The facility is "participating" under Medicare law. Hospital Insurance will not pay for a person's stay if he needs skilled nursing or rehabilitation services only occasionally, such as once or twice a week, or if a person does not need to be in a skilled nursing facility to obtain skilled rehabilitation services. And, Hospital Insurance will not pay for a person's stay if the rehabilitation services are no longer improving his condition and could be carried out by someone other than a physical therapist or physical therapist assistant.

HOME HEALTH CARE

B-31. When are post-hospital home health services covered under Hospital Insurance?

If a person needs post-institutional skilled health care in his home for the treatment of an illness or injury, Medicare pays for covered home health services furnished by a participating home health agency. Hospital Insurance covers the cost of 100 home health visits made on an "intermittent" basis during a home health spell of illness under a plan of treatment established by a physician.

A "home health agency" is a public agency or private organization which

(1) is primarily engaged in providing skilled nursing services and other therapeutic services,

(2) has policies, established by a group of professional personnel, including one or more physicians and one or more registered professional nurses, to govern the services which it provides, and provides for supervision of its services by a physician or registered professional nurse,

(3) maintains clinical records on all patients,

(4) is licensed pursuant to applicable state and local law,

(5) has in effect an overall plan and budget,

(6) meets additional requirements and conditions of participation as the Department of Health and Human Services finds necessary in the interest of the health and safety of individuals who are furnished services by the home health agency,

(7) meets additional requirements of the Department of Health and Human Services for the effective and efficient operation of the program.

A "home health agency" does not include any agency or organization which is primarily for the care and treatment of mental diseases.

A number of rules and procedures have been established to stop fraud and abuse, including regulations requiring all home health agencies serving Medicare to obtain surety bonds. Agencies must be bonded and must provide quality care to at least 10 patients before applying to provide care to Medicare patients. At least seven of the 10 patients must be receiving active care at the time the agency applies for entry into Medicare.

B-32. What conditions must be met for Hospital Insurance to cover home health visits?

Hospital Insurance pays for the first 100 home health visits in a "home health spell of illness" if all six of the following conditions are met:

(1) The care is post-institutional home health services.

(2) The care includes intermittent skilled nursing care, physical therapy, or speech therapy.

(3) The person is confined at home.

(4) The person is under the care of a physician who determines the need for home health care and sets up a home health plan for the person.

(5) The home health agency providing services participates in Medicare.

(6) The services are provided on a visiting basis in the person's home, or if it is necessary to use equipment that cannot be readily made available in the home, on an outpatient basis in a hospital, skilled nursing facility, or licensed rehabilitation center.

The term "post-institutional home health services" means home health services furnished to an individual

(1) After discharge from a hospital or rural primary care hospital in which the individual was an inpatient for at least three consecutive days before discharge. Home health services must be initiated within 14 days after the date of discharge.

(2) After discharge from a skilled nursing facility in which the individual was provided post-hospital extended care services. Home health services must be initiated within 14 days after the date of discharge.

The term "home health spell of illness" means a period of consecutive days (1) beginning with the first day a person is furnished post-institutional home health services (in a month in which the person is entitled to benefits under Part A), and (2) ending with the close of the first period of 60 consecutive days thereafter for which the person is neither an inpatient in a hospital or skilled nursing facility nor provided home health services.

"Part-time or intermittent services" is defined as skilled nursing and home health aid services (combined) furnished any number of days per week, for less than eight hours per day and 28 or fewer hours per week (or, subject to review on a case-by-case basis as to the need for care, less than eight hours each day and 35 or fewer hours per week).

"Intermittent" is defined as skilled nursing care provided on fewer than seven days each week, or less than eight hours each day (combined) for 21 days or less (with extensions in exceptional circumstances when the need for additional care is finite and predictable).

A doctor must certify that the person is under a doctor's care, under a plan of care established and periodically reviewed no less frequently than every two months by a doctor, confined to the home, and in need of (1) skilled nursing care on an intermittent basis, or (2) physical or speech therapy, or has a continued need for (3) occupational therapy when eligibility for home health services has been established because of a prior need for intermittent skilled nursing care, speech therapy, or physical therapy in the current or prior certification period.

Home health aides, whether employed directly by a home health agency or made available through contract with another entity, must successfully complete a training and competency evaluation program or competency evaluation program approved by the Department of Health and Human Services.

Generally, a doctor may not set up a home health care plan for a patient with any agency in which the doctor has a significant ownership interest or a significant financial or contractual relationship. But a doctor who has a financial interest in an agency which is a sole community health agency may carry out certification and plan of care functions for patients served by that agency.

B-33. What post-hospital home health services are covered under Hospital Insurance?

The following post-hospital home health services are covered under Hospital Insurance:

- Part-time or intermittent skilled nursing care. (See B-32.)

- Physical therapy.

- Speech therapy.

If a person needs part-time or intermittent skilled nursing care, physical therapy, or speech therapy, Medicare also pays for

- Part-time or intermittent services of home health aides. Covered services include, but are not limited to (1) personal care, (2) simple dressing changes that do not require the skills of a licensed nurse, (3) assistance with medications that are ordinarily self-administered and that do not require a licensed nurse, (4) assistance with activities supportive of skilled therapy services, and (5) routine care of prosthetic devices.

- Medical social services.

- Medical supplies, including catheters, catheter supplies, ostomy bags, and ostomy care supplies.

- Durable medical equipment (80% of approved cost), including iron lungs, oxygen tents, hospital beds, and wheelchairs.

- Occupational therapy.

The patient pays nothing for the first 100 home health visits. Medicare pays the full approved cost of all covered home health visits. The patient may be charged only for any services or costs that Medicare does not cover. However, if the patient needs durable medical equipment, the patient is responsible for a 20% coinsurance payment for the equipment. The home health agency will submit claims for payment. The patient does not send in any bills.

Both Hospital Insurance (Part A) and Medical Insurance (Part B) cover home health visits, but Hospital Insurance pays for the first 100 visits following a hospital or skilled nursing facility stay while Medical Insurance only pays for home health services that are unassociated with a hospital or skilled nursing facility stay.

Medicare does not cover home care services furnished primarily to assist people in meeting personal, family, and domestic needs. These non-covered services include general household services such as laundry, meal preparation, shopping, or assisting in bathing, dressing, or other personal needs.

Home health services *not* covered by Medicare also include

- 24-hour-a-day nursing care at home,

- drugs and biologicals,

- blood transfusions,

- meals delivered to the home,

- homemaker services, and

- venipuncture (drawing of blood for the purpose of obtaining a blood sample), if venipuncture is the only skilled service needed by the beneficiary.

While the patient must be homebound to be eligible for benefits, payment will be made for services furnished at a hospital, skilled nursing facility, or rehabilitation center if the patient's condition requires the use of equipment that ordinarily cannot be taken to the patient's home. However, Medicare will not pay the patient's transportation costs.

A patient is considered "confined to the home" if he or she has a condition, due to illness or injury, that restricts the ability to leave home except with the assistance of another person or the aid of a supportive device (such as crutches, a cane, a wheelchair, or a walker), or if the patient has a condition such that leaving home is medically unsafe. While a patient does not have to be bedridden to be considered "confined to the home," the condition should be such that there exists a normal inability to leave home, that leaving home requires a considerable and taxing effort, and that absences from home are infrequent or of relatively short duration, or are attributable to the need to receive medical treatment.

Infrequent means an average of five or fewer absences per calendar month, excluding absences to receive medical treatment that cannot be furnished in the home. *Short duration* means an average of three or fewer hours per absence from the home within a calendar month, excluding absences to receive medical treatment that cannot be furnished in the home. Absences for medical treatment must be (1) based on and in conformance with a physician's order, (2) by or under the supervision of a licensed health professional, and (3) for the purpose of diagnosis or treatment of an illness or injury.

The *Home Health Agency Manual* of the Centers for Medicare & Medicaid Services provides examples of patients qualifying as homebound. They include (1) a person paralyzed from a stroke who is confined to a wheelchair and who requires crutches in order to walk, (2) a person who is blind or senile and requires the assistance of another person in leaving his residence, (3) a person who has lost the use of upper extremities and is unable to open doors, use stairways, etc., and, therefore, requires the assistance of another person to leave his residence, and (4) a person with a psychiatric problem if the person's illness is manifested in part by a refusal to leave his home environment, or is of such a nature that it would not be considered safe for the patient to leave home unattended, even if the patient has no physical limitations.

Home health agencies are required to provide patients with the following rights: (1) the right to be informed of and to participate in planning care and treatment, (2) the right to confidentiality of clinical records, (3) the right to voice grievances, (4) the right to advance notice, including notice in writing, of items and services for which payment will and will not be paid by Medicare, (5) the right to have property treated with respect, (6) the right to be fully informed in advance of Medicare rights and obligations, and (7) the right to be informed of the availability of a state Home Health Agency Hot Line.

B-34. How does Medicare pay the costs of home health services?

The Centers for Medicare & Medicaid Services has established a prospective payment system for all costs of home health services. In defining a payment amount under a prospective payment system, the Centers for Medicare & Medicaid Services considers an appropriate unit of service and the number, type, and duration of visits provided within that unit of service. The Centers for Medicare & Medicaid Services also considers potential changes in the mix of services provided within a unit and their cost. The general design of a unit of service is to provide for continued access to quality services. All bills for service must be submitted by the home health agency for payment and not by any other person or entity.

Prospective payment amounts are to be standardized in a manner that eliminates the effect of variations in relative case mix and wage levels among different home health agencies in a budget neutral manner. Under the system, the Centers for Medicare & Medicaid Services may recognize regional differences or differences based upon whether the services or agencies are in an urbanized area. The standard prospective payment amount (or amounts) is adjusted for each fiscal year.

GENERAL INFORMATION

B-35. Does Hospital Insurance (Part A) pay the cost of outpatient hospital services?

No. Outpatient diagnostic and treatment services are covered under Medical Insurance (Part B). (See SECTION C.)

B-36. Does a person need to be in financial need to receive Hospital Insurance benefits?

No. Benefits are not subject to any means testing.

B-37. Will the deductible and coinsurance amounts paid by patients remain the same in future years?

No. The $992 initial deductible for inpatient hospital care for 2007 is based on the 1966-68 figure of $40 and increases in average per diem inpatient hospital cost since 1966 (and also some legislative changes) and, beginning with the 1987 determination, on increases in average national hospital costs, based on a hospital-cost "market basket" index. The daily coinsurance amounts are based on this per diem rate. The daily coinsurance for inpatient hospital care for the 61st through 90th days in a benefit period is 1/4 of the initial deductible ($248 in 2007). The daily coinsurance for post-hospital extended care after 20 days is 1/8 of this initial deductible ($124.00 in 2007). The lifetime reserve days' coinsurance is 1/2 of the initial deductible ($496 in 2007).

B-38. What is Medicare's position regarding treatment of a patient with a living will or durable power of attorney for health care?

The Centers for Medicare & Medicaid Services has regulations that require all hospitals, skilled nursing facilities, nursing facilities, providers of home health care or personal care services, hospices, and prepaid health plans to provide the patient with written information concerning rights under state law to make decisions concerning medical care, including the right to accept or refuse medical or surgical treatment and the right to formulate, at the patient's option, advance directives. The regulations do not apply to providers of outpatient hospital services.

The term "advance directive" is defined as a written instrument, such as a living will or durable power of attorney for health care, recognized under state law, relating to the provision of health care when the individual is incapacitated. The individual is not required to execute an advance directive prior to the start of treatment or services under Medicare.

The provider must (1) inform the individual, in writing, of state laws regarding advance directives, (2) inform the individual, in writing, of the policies of the provider regarding the implementation of advance directives, including if permitted under state law, a clear and precise explanation of any objection a provider may have, on the basis of conscience, to honoring an individual's directive, (3) document in the individual's medical record whether or not the individual has executed an advance directive, (4) educate staff on issues concerning advance directives, and (5) provide for community education on issues concerning advance directives.

Providers must communicate information to individuals about their right to accept or refuse medical treatment and the right to formulate an advance directive by furnishing written descriptions of state law and provider policies and practices regarding the implementation of such rights.

Written information on advance directives must be provided to an individual upon each admission to a medical facility and each time an individual comes under the care of a home health agency, personal care provider, or hospice. For example, if a person is admitted first as an inpatient to a hospital and then to a nursing home, both the hospital and the nursing home are required to provide information on advance directives to the individual. If the patient is incapacitated at the time of admission and is unable to receive information or articulate whether or not an advance directive has been executed, the facility may give advance directive information to the patient's family or surrogate.

All patients are generally entitled to the medically necessary care ordered by a physician which a provider, under normal procedures, would be required to furnish and cannot delay or withhold because the individual has not executed an advance directive or the provider is waiting for an advance directive to be executed. However, once it is documented that an advance directive has been executed, then the directive takes precedence over the facility's normal procedures, to the extent required by state law.

A health care provider is not required to implement an advance directive if, as a matter of conscience, the provider cannot implement an advance directive and state law allows any health care provider to conscientiously object. The provider must inform individuals that complaints concerning non-compliance with the advance directive requirements may be filed with the state survey and certification agency.

PART B:

MEDICAL INSURANCE

ELIGIBILITY

C-1. Who is eligible for Medical Insurance benefits?

All persons entitled to premium-free Hospital Insurance (Part A), or premium Hospital Insurance (Part A) for the working disabled under Medicare, may enroll in Medical Insurance (Part B). Social Security and Railroad Retirement beneficiaries, age 65 or over, are, therefore, automatically eligible. But any other person age 65 or over may enroll provided that he is a resident of the United States and is either (1) a citizen of the United States or (2) an alien lawfully admitted for permanent residence who has resided in the United States continuously during the five years immediately prior to the month in which he applies for enrollment.

Disabled beneficiaries (workers under age 65, widows aged 50-64, and children aged 18 or over disabled before age 22) who have been on the benefit roll as a disability beneficiary for at least two years are covered in the same manner as persons age 65 or over. (This includes disabled railroad retirement beneficiaries.) Disability cases are also covered for 48 months after cash benefits cease for a worker who is engaging in substantial gainful employment but has not medically recovered. (Disability benefits are, under such circumstances, paid for the first nine months of the trial-work period and then for an additional three months.) After 48 months, and during continued disability, voluntary coverage is available in the same manner as for non-insured persons age 65 or over.

A person can continue to buy Medicare (Hospital Insurance (Part A) only or both Hospital Insurance and Medical Insurance (Part B)) as long as he remains disabled. Such a person may enroll during his initial enrollment period which begins with the month the person is notified he is no longer eligible for premium-free Hospital Insurance and continues for seven full months after that month. If a person does not enroll during this initial enrollment period, the person may enroll in a subsequent general enrollment period (January through March of each year) or during a special enrollment period.

Also covered are persons with end-stage renal disease who require dialysis or a kidney transplant and are eligible for Hospital Insurance (Part A).

C-2. How does a person enroll in Medical Insurance?

Those who are receiving Social Security and Railroad Retirement benefits will be enrolled automatically at the time they become entitled to Hospital Insurance unless they elect not to be covered for Medical Insurance by signing a form which will be sent to them. Others may enroll at their nearest Social Security office.

The initial enrollment period is a period of seven full calendar months, the beginning and end of which is determined for each person by the day on which he is first eligible to enroll. The initial enrollment period begins on the first day of the third month before the month a person first becomes eligible to enroll and ends with the close of the last day of the third month following the month a person first becomes eligible to enroll. For example, if the person's 65th birthday is April 10, 2007, the initial enrollment period begins January 1, 2007 and ends July 31, 2007.

If a person decides not to enroll in the initial enrollment period, he may enroll during a special enrollment period. (See C-3.) The special enrollment period is a period provided by statute to enable certain individuals to enroll in Medicare without waiting for the general enrollment period.

In order to obtain coverage at the earliest possible date, a person must enroll before the beginning of the month in which age 65 is reached. For a person who enrolls during the initial enrollment period, the effective date of coverage is as follows:

(1) If the person enrolls before the month in which age 65 is reached, coverage will commence the first day of the month in which age 65 is reached.

(2) If the person enrolls during the month in which age 65 is reached, coverage will commence the first day of the following month.

(3) If the person enrolls in the month after the month in which age 65 is reached, coverage will commence the first day of the second month after the month of enrollment.

(4) If the person enrolls more than one month (but at least within three months) after the month in which age 65 is reached, coverage will commence the first day of the third month following the month of enrollment.

A seven-month special enrollment period is provided if Medicare has been the secondary payer of benefits for individuals age 65 and older who are covered under an employer group health plan because of current employment. The special enrollment period generally begins with the month in which coverage under the private plan ends. Coverage under Medical Insurance (Part B) will begin with the month after coverage under the private plan ends, if the individual enrolls in that month, or with the month after enrollment, if the individual enrolls during the balance of the special enrollment period. (See C-3.)

C-3. What if a person declines to enroll during the automatic enrollment period?

Anyone who fails to enroll during the initial enrollment period may enroll during a general enrollment period. There are general enrollment periods each year from January 1st through March 31st. Coverage begins the following July 1st.

The premium will be higher for a person who fails to enroll within 12 months, or who drops out of the plan and later re-enrolls. The monthly premium will be increased by 10% for each full 12 months during which he could have been, but was not, enrolled.

If a person declines to enroll (or terminates enrollment) at a time when Medicare is secondary payer to his employer group health plan, the months in which he is covered under the employer group health plan (based on current employment) and Hospital

Insurance will not be counted as months during which he could have been but was not enrolled in Medical Insurance for the purpose of determining if the premium amount should be increased above the basic rate. These people may then enroll during the "special enrollment period." The special enrollment period lasts for seven months and starts the first month the person is not covered by a group health plan.

Individuals must meet the following conditions to enroll during the special enrollment period:

(1) They must be eligible for Medical Insurance (Part B) on the basis of age or disability, but not on the basis of end-stage renal disease.

(2) When first eligible for Medical Insurance coverage (fourth month of their initial enrollment period), they must be covered under a group health plan or large group health plan on the basis of current employment status or, if not so covered, they must enroll in Medical Insurance during their initial enrollment period.

(3) For all months thereafter, they must maintain coverage under either Medical Insurance or a group health plan or large group health plan. (Generally, if an individual fails to enroll in Medical Insurance during any available special enrollment period, he is not entitled to any additional special enrollment periods. However, if an individual fails to enroll during a special enrollment period because coverage under the same or a different group health plan or large group health plan was restored before the end of that particular special enrollment period, that failure to enroll does not preclude additional special enrollment periods.)

A large group health plan is a plan of an employer with 100 or more employees or of a group of employers at least one of which has 100 or more employees.

For an individual who is or was covered under a group health plan, coverage must be by reason of the current employment status of the individual or the individual's spouse.

Individuals entitled on the basis of disability (but not end-stage renal disease) must meet conditions that vary depending on whether they were covered under a group health plan or a large group health plan.

C-4. Can a person be enrolled under a federal-state/local agreement?

Upon the request of an appropriate state or local government entity, the Department of Health and Human Services may enter into an agreement whereby the state or local government entity agrees to pay, on a quarterly or other periodic basis, an amount equal to the total Part B late enrollment surcharge amounts for a group of individuals chosen by the state or local government.

C-5. Is there a special enrollment period for disabled workers who lose benefits under a group health plan?

Certain disabled beneficiaries are eligible for a special enrollment period and waiver of the Part B premium surcharge. These individuals are disabled beneficiaries (1) who were enrolled in a group health plan (by reason of current or former employment or the current or former employment of a family member) at the time of initially becoming eligible for Medicare, (2) who elected not to enroll in Part B during their initial enrollment period, and (3) whose continuous enrollment under the group health plan is involuntarily terminated at a time when the enrollment is by reason of the individual's former employment (or the former employment of a family member).

The special enrollment period begins on the first day of the month that includes the date of the involuntary termination and continues for six months.

C-6. How does a person terminate or cancel coverage?

A person's coverage period continues until his enrollment is terminated. A beneficiary can terminate coverage by filing a notice that he no longer wishes to participate in the program. He can also terminate coverage by not paying the monthly premium.

The termination of coverage takes effect at the close of the month following the month in which the notice is filed. A grace period is provided before coverage is terminated for not paying premiums. The grace period in which overdue premiums can be paid and coverage continued may not exceed 90 days (180 days in cases where the Department of Health and Human Services determines that there was good cause for failure to pay the overdue premiums within the 90-day period).

A termination notice filed by a person enrolled in Medical Insurance before the first day of the month that coverage begins will terminate coverage on the first day of the month in which coverage would have been effective. If a termination notice is filed in or after the month in which coverage is effective, the coverage is terminated at the close of the month following the month in which the notice is filed.

In the case of a person entitled to Hospital Insurance based on 24 or more months of disability, rather than on having attained age 65, Medical Insurance is terminated at the close of the last month for which he is entitled to Hospital Insurance benefits.

FINANCING MEDICAL INSURANCE

C-7. How is Medical Insurance (Part B) financed?

Medical Insurance is voluntary and is financed through premiums paid by people who enroll and through funds from the federal government. These monthly premiums are in addition to the deductible and coinsurance amounts that must be paid by the patient.

Most persons enrolled pay a standard monthly premium of $93.50 per month in 2007. The basic Medical Insurance premium is set to cover 25% of program costs each year. The federal government pays the remaining cost from general revenues. In September-October of each year, the Centers for Medicare & Medicaid Services announces the premium rate for the 12-month period starting the following January.

Beginning in 2007, single persons with annual incomes over $80,000 and married couples with incomes over $160,000 will pay a higher percentage of the cost of Medicare Insurance. These higher-income beneficiaries will pay a monthly premium equal to 35%, 50%, 65%, or 80% of the total cost, depending on their income level, by the end of the

3-year transition period. For 2007, the higher-income beneficiaries will be responsible for one-third of the income-related monthly adjustment amount.

The premium rate for a person who enrolls after the first period when enrollment is open, or who re-enrolls after terminating coverage, will be increased by 10% for each full 12 months the person stayed out of the program.

Basic Monthly Premium
Medical Insurance

Year	Monthly Premium
1986	$15.50
1987	17.90
1988	24.80
1989	27.90
1990	28.60
1991	29.90
1992	31.80
1993	36.60
1994	41.10
1995	46.10
1996	42.50
1997	43.80
1998	43.80
1999	45.50
2000	45.50
2001	50.00
2002	54.00
2003	58.70
2004	66.60
2005	78.20
2006	88.50
2007	93.50

Income-Adjusted Monthly Premium
Medical Insurance

Single Taxpayer	Married Taxpayers Filing Jointly	Total Premium
Not greater than $80,000	Not greater than $160,000	$93.50
$80,001 - $100,000	$160,001 - $200,000	105.80
$100,001 - $150,000	$200,001 - $300,000	124.40
$150,001 - $200,000	$300,001 - $400,000	142.90
$200,001 and up	$400,001 and up	161.40

Married Taxpayers Separately	Total Premium
Not greater than $80,000	$93.50
$80,001 - $120,000	142.90
$120,001 and up	161.40

C-8. What is a Qualified Medicare Beneficiary?

An elderly or disabled person with a low income who is eligible for Medicare may be able to have some or all Medicare expenses paid by their state. Federal law requires state Medicaid programs to pay Medicare costs for certain elderly and disabled persons with low incomes and very limited assets.

There are three programs to help people pay their Medicare expenses. One is called the "Qualified Medicare Beneficiary" or "QMB" program. Another is called the "Specified Low-Income Medicare Beneficiary" or "SLMB" program. The final program is called the "Qualifying Individual" or "QI" program.

The QMB program is for persons with limited resources whose incomes are at or below the national poverty level. It covers the cost of Medicare premiums, coinsurance and deductibles that Medicare beneficiaries normally pay out of their own pockets. The QMB program also pays the basic Medical Insurance (Part B) premium, which is $93.50 a month in 2007.

While the QMB program helps those whose income is at or below the national poverty level, the SLMB program is for persons whose incomes are slightly higher than the poverty level, but not more than 20% higher. The state pays the Medical Insurance premium ($93.50 in 2007) for a person qualifying under the SLMB program. However, the person remains responsible for Medicare's deductibles, coinsurance, and for charges for health care services and medical supplies not covered by Medicare.

The QI Program assists individuals and married couples whose income is more than 20% greater than the Federal poverty level, but not more than 35% greater in order to have the full monthly Medical Insurance (Part B) premium paid each month ("QI-1"). The "QI-2" program, which paid a small portion of the monthly Medical Insurance (Part B) premium paid each month, was not re-authorized after 2002. Persons covered under the QI Program remain responsible for Medicare's deductibles and coinsurance and for charges for health care services and medical supplies not covered by Medicare (and, if applicable, the majority of the monthly Medical Insurance (Part B) premiums).

The rules vary from state to state but, in general terms, to qualify for assistance under the QMB program, a person must meet the following requirements:

(1) The person must be entitled to Hospital Insurance (Part A).

(2) The person's financial resources such as bank accounts, stocks, and bonds cannot exceed $4,000 for one person or $6,000 for a couple. Some things—the home the person lives in, one automobile, burial plots, home furnishings, personal jewelry, and life insurance—usually do not count as resources.

(3) The person's income must be at or below the national poverty level. The QMB annual income limits in 2007 (until adjusted no later than April 1, 2007) are $9,804 for an individual, and $13,200 for a couple. Income includes, but is not limited to, Social Security benefits, pensions and wages. Interest payments and dividends can also count as income.

If a person does not qualify for QMB assistance because his income is too high, he may be able to get help under the SLMB program. To qualify for SLMB assistance, a person must meet requirements (1) and (2) listed above. Also, a person's income cannot exceed the national poverty level by more than 20%. This means that in 2007 (until adjusted no later than April 1, 2007) the SLMB annual income limits are $11,760 annually for an individual, and $15,840 annually for a couple. The 2007 amounts (until adjusted no later than April 1, 2007) for the QI Program are an annual maximum of $13.236 for an individual or $17,820 for a couple for QI-1 assistance.

If a person already has Medicare Part A and thinks he may qualify for QMB, SLMB, or QI assistance, he must file an application for assistance at a state, county, or local medical assistance office.

C-9. How are premiums paid under Medical Insurance?

Persons covered have the premiums deducted from their Social Security, Railroad Retirement, or federal civil service retirement benefit checks. Persons who are not receiving any of these government benefits pay the premiums directly to the government.

Direct payment of premiums is usually made on a quarterly basis with a grace period, determined by the Department of Health and Human Services, of up to 90 days.

Public assistance agencies may enroll, and pay premiums for, public assistance recipients (Supplemental Security Income program). States must pay premiums for specified low-income persons. (See C-8.)

If a person's Social Security or Railroad Retirement benefits are suspended because of excess earnings, and benefits will not be resumed until the next taxable year, the person will be billed directly for overdue Medicare premiums. If Social Security or Railroad Retirement benefits will be resumed before the close of the taxable year, overdue premiums are deducted from the Social Security or Railroad Retirement cash benefits when they resume.

Premiums must be paid for the entire month of death even though coverage ends on the day of death.

C-10. How are "approved charges" for covered medical services determined?

There are three major elements that determine how much Medicare pays for physician services: (1) a fee schedule for the payment of physician services, (2) a method to control the rates of increase in Medicare expenditures for physicians' services, and (3) limits on the amounts that nonparticipating physicians can charge beneficiaries. Payments under the fee schedule must be based on national uniform relative value units (RVUs) based on the resources used in furnishing a service. National RVUs must be established for physician work, practice expense, and malpractice expense.

Adjustments in RVUs because of changes resulting from a review of those RVUs may not cause total physician fee schedule payments to differ by more than $20 million from what they would have been had the adjustments not been made. If this amount is exceeded, the Centers for Medicare & Medicaid Services must make an adjustment to the conversion factor to preserve budget neutrality.

The Centers for Medicare & Medicaid Services is required to review and, if necessary, adjust the geographic practice cost indices (GPCIs) at least every three years. It also must phase in the adjustment over two years and implement only one-half of any adjustment if more than one year has elapsed since the last GPCI revision.

Payments must vary among fee schedule areas according to geographic indices.

C-11. How are Medical Insurance (Part B) payments made?

Medical Insurance payments are made in two ways. Payment can be made directly to the doctor or supplier. This is the assignment method of payment. Payment can also be made to the patient.

Under the assignment method, the doctor or supplier agrees to accept the amount approved by the Medicare carrier as total payment for covered services.

The assignment method can save the patient time and money. The doctor or supplier sends the claim to Medicare. Medicare pays the doctor or supplier 80% of the Medicare-approved charge, after subtracting any part of the annual deductible ($131 for 2007) the patient has not paid. The doctor or supplier can charge the patient *only* for the part of the annual deductible he has not met and for the coinsurance, which is the remaining 20% of the approved amount. Of course, a doctor or supplier also can charge the patient for any services that Medicare does not cover.

If a doctor does not accept assignment (nonparticipating physician), Medicare pays the patient 80% of the approved charge, after subtracting any part of the annual deductible the patient has not paid. The doctor or supplier can bill the patient for his actual charge even if it is more than the charge approved by the Medicare carrier.

Doctors, suppliers and other providers of Medical Insurance (Part B) services are in most cases required to submit Medicare claims for the patient, even if they do not take assignment. The doctor or supplier must submit a form, called a CMS-1500, requesting that Medical Insurance payment be made for a patient's covered services. The doctor or supplier completes the form and the patient signs it before it is sent to the proper Medicare carrier. The doctor or supplier must submit a claim within one year of providing the service or may be subject to certain penalties. A patient should notify the Medicare carrier if a doctor or supplier refuses to submit a Medical Insurance claim and the patient believes the services may be covered by Medicare.

If a patient is enrolled in a prepaid health care organization such as an HMO, a claim will seldom need to be submitted. Medicare pays the HMO a set amount and the HMO provides medical care for its members. Doctors, suppliers and other providers of Medical Insurance (Part B) services bill the HMO directly for reimbursement at contractually-agreed rates.

Utilizing a doctor who accepts assignment under Medicare can make a big difference in a patient's out-of-pocket costs.

Example. Jane Smith has surgery after meeting the annual deductible for Medical Insurance. Dr. Ralph Jones, who is not a participating physician and does not limit his charges to the Medicare fee schedule, bills Ms. Smith $1,200 for the surgery. The Medicare fee schedule sets the charge for this surgery at $1,100. Medicare will pay $880 (80% of the Medicare fee) and Ms. Smith must pay the remaining $320 of the $1,200 fee.

If Dr. Jones had been a participating physician under Medicare, Ms. Smith would have had to pay only $220 (20% of the approved charge of $1,100 that Medicare does not pay).

If a physician does not accept the assignment method, he must refund all amounts collected from Medicare beneficiaries on claims for services that are deemed not medically necessary. The Medicare carrier will send a notice to the beneficiary and physician advising them of the basis for denial, the right of appeal, and the requirement of a refund.

Even though a doctor does not accept assignment, for most covered services there are limits on the amount he can actually charge the patient. The most a doctor can charge is 115% of what Medicare approves. The 115% limit also applies to fees for physical and occupational therapy services, suppliers, injections, and other services billable under the physician fee schedule.

Physicians must give written notice prior to elective surgery for which the fee is $500 or more. The notice must state the physician's estimated actual charge, the estimated Medicare-approved charge, the excess of the actual charge over the approved charge, and the applicable coinsurance amount. This requirement applies to non-emergency surgical procedures only. (Emergency surgery is surgery performed under conditions and circumstances which afford no alternatives to the physician or the patient and, if delayed, could result in death or permanent impairment of health.) If the physician fails to make this fee disclosure, and the surgery was non-emergency surgery, the physician must refund amounts collected in excess of the Medicare-approved Medical Insurance (Part B) charge. The physician is subject to sanctions if he knowingly and willfully fails to comply with this refund requirement.

C-12. How can a person find out if a doctor accepts assignment of all Medicare claims?

Doctors and suppliers sign agreements in advance to accept assignment on all Medicare claims. They are given the opportunity to sign participation agreements each year.

The names and addresses of Medicare-participating doctors are listed by geographic area in the *Medicare-Participating Physician Directory*. This directory is available free of charge from the Medicare carrier, and a person can call the Medicare carrier for the names of some participating doctors and suppliers in the area. The names and addresses of Medicare participating suppliers are listed by geographic area in the *Medicare-Participating Supplier Directory*. This directory is available by calling the Durable Medical Equipment Regional Carrier in the area. Both directories are also available in Social Security offices, state and area offices of the Administration on Aging, most hospitals, and at www.medicare.gov.

Medicare-participating doctors and suppliers may display emblems or certificates that show they accept assignment on all Medicare claims.

C-13. What are Medicare providers and Medicare suppliers?

The term "provider" means a hospital, a rural primary care hospital, a skilled nursing facility, a comprehensive outpatient rehabilitative facility, a home health agency, or a hospice that has in effect an agreement to participate in Medicare. A clinic, rehabilitation agency, or a public health agency that has a similar agreement to furnish outpatient physical therapy or speech pathology services, or a community mental health center with a similar agreement to furnish partial hospitalization services, is also considered a provider.

In general, "suppliers" are individuals or entities, other than doctors or health care facilities, that furnish equipment or services covered by Medical Insurance. For example, ambulance firms, independent laboratories, and entities that rent or sell medical equipment are considered suppliers.

There are different definitions of the term supplier and specific regulations governing different types of suppliers. Durable medical equipment, prosthetics, orthotics, and supplies (DMEPOS) encompasses the types of items included in the definition of "medical equipment and supplies." A "DMEPOS supplier" refers to all individuals or organizations that furnish these items. This can include a physician or Medicare Part A provider. A DMEPOS supplier must meet Medicare DMEPOS standards in order to obtain a supplier number. Those individuals or entities that do not furnish DMEPOS items but only furnish other types of health care services, such as physician's services or nurse practitioner services, are not subject to these standards. A supplier number is also not necessary before Medicare payment can be made with respect to medical equipment and supplies furnished incident to a physician's service.

For Medicare purposes, DMEPOS suppliers either accept or do not accept assignment. If a DMEPOS supplier accepts assignment, it agrees to accept the Medicare approved amount as payment in full for the covered item. They are referred to as "participating suppliers." Participating DMEPOS suppliers are listed in directories available to Medicare beneficiaries and receive Medicare Part B payment directly from the Medicare program. Nonparticipating DMEPOS suppliers may accept assignment on a case-by-case basis, and for these claims, receive payment directly from Medicare. If a beneficiary receives a service from a nonparticipating DMEPOS supplier on a nonassigned basis, however, payment is made to the beneficiary who in turn pays the DMEPOS supplier.

A supplier is required to meet 11 standards including the following: (1) complying with all applicable state and federal license and regulatory requirements, (2) maintaining a physical facility on an appropriate site, (3) having proof of appropriate liability insurance, (4) delivering Medicare covered items to Medicare beneficiaries, (5) honoring all warranties, (6) maintaining and repairing items rented to beneficiaries, and (7) accepting returns of substandard or unsuitable items from beneficiaries.

C-14. What portion of the cost must be borne by the patient?

The patient pays the first $131 of covered expenses incurred in calendar year 2007. Medicare pays 80% of the balance of the approved charges (50% generally for out-of-hospital psychiatric services) over the annual deductible. But there is no cost-sharing for most home health services, pneumococcal vaccine, flu shot, the costs of second opinions for certain surgical procedures when Medicare requires these opinions, and outpatient clinical diagnostic laboratory tests performed by hospitals and independent laboratories which are Medicare-certified and by physicians who accept assignment.

C-15. How does a patient find out how much Medicare will pay on a claim?

After the doctor, provider, or supplier sends in a Medical Insurance claim, Medicare sends the patient a notice called *Explanation of Your Medicare Part B Benefits* to tell the patient the decision on the claim.

This notice shows what charges were made and what Medicare approved. It shows what the coinsurance is and what Medicare is paying. If the annual deductible had not been met, that is also shown. The notice also gives the address and telephone number of the carrier.

BENEFITS

C-16. What doctors' services are covered under Medical Insurance (Part B)?

Under Medical Insurance, Medicare usually pays 80% of the approved charges for doctors' services and the cost of other services that are covered under Medical Insurance after the patient pays annual deductible. Medical Insurance helps pay for covered services received from the doctor in the doctor's office, in a hospital, in a skilled nursing facility, in the patient's home, or any other location. The following doctors' fees and services are covered by Medical Insurance:

- *Doctors' services* are covered wherever furnished in the United States. This includes the cost of house calls, office visits, and doctors' services in a hospital or other institution. It includes the fees of physicians, surgeons, pathologists, radiologists, anesthesiologists, physiatrists, and osteopaths.

- Services from certain *specially qualified practitioners* who are not physicians but are approved by Medicare, including certified registered nurse anesthetists, certified nurse midwifes, clinical psychologists, clinical social workers (other than in a hospital), physician assistants, and nurse practitioners and clinical nurse specialists in collaboration with a physician.

- Services of *clinical psychologists* are covered if they would otherwise be covered when furnished by a physician (or as an incident to a physician's services).

- Services by *licensed chiropractors* for manual manipulation of the spine to correct a subluxation. Medical Insurance does not pay for any other diagnostic or therapeutic services, including X-rays, furnished by a chiropractor. Medicare pays for manual manipulation of the spine to correct a subluxation without requiring an X-ray (which previously was required) to prove that the subluxation exists.

- Fees of *podiatrists* are covered, including fees for the treatment of plantar warts, but not for routine foot care. Examples of common problems covered by Medical

Insurance include ingrown toenails, hammer toe deformities, bunion deformities, and heel spurs. Routine foot care not covered by Medical Insurance includes cutting or removal of corns and calluses, trimming of nails, and other hygienic care. Medical Insurance does help pay for some routine foot care if the patient is being treated by a medical doctor for a medical condition affecting the patient's legs or feet (such as diabetes or peripheral vascular disease) which requires that a podiatrist or doctor of medicine or osteopathy perform the routine care. The cost of treatment of debridement of mycotic toenails (i.e., the care of toenails with a fungal infection) is not included if performed more frequently than once every 60 days. Exceptions are authorized if medical necessity is documented by the billing physician.

Medicare helps pay for therapeutic shoes and shoe inserts for people who have severe diabetic foot disease. The doctor who treats the diabetes must certify the patient's need for therapeutic shoes. The shoes and inserts must be prescribed by a podiatrist and furnished by a podiatrist, orthotist, prosthetist, or pedorthist. Medicare helps pay for one pair of therapeutic shoes per calendar year and for inserts. Shoe modifications may be substituted for inserts. The fitting of shoes or inserts is included in the Medicare payment for the shoes.

- The cost of diagnosis and treatment of *eye and ear ailments* is covered. Also covered is an *optometrist's treatment of aphakia*.

- *Plastic surgery* for purely cosmetic reasons is excluded; but plastic surgery for repair of an accidental injury, an impaired limb or a malformed part of the body is covered.

- *Radiological or pathological services* furnished by a physician to a hospital inpatient are covered.

Medical Insurance covers (1) medical and surgical services, including anesthesia, (2) diagnostic tests and procedures that are part of the patient's treatment, (3) radiology and pathology services by doctors while the patient is a hospital inpatient or outpatient, (4) treatment of mental illness (Medicare payments are limited), (5) X-rays, (6) services of the doctor's office nurse, (7) drugs and biologicals that cannot be self-administered, (8) transfusions of blood and blood components, (9) medical supplies, and (10) physical/occupational therapy and speech-language pathology services.

Medical Insurance does *not* cover (1) most routine physical examinations, and tests directly related to such examinations (except some Pap smears and mammograms), (2) most routine foot care and dental care, (3) examinations for prescribing or fitting eyeglasses or hearing aids and most eyeglasses and hearing aids, (4) immunizations (except annual flu shots, pneumococcal pneumonia vaccinations or immunizations required because of an injury or immediate risk of infection, and hepatitis B for certain persons at risk), (5) cosmetic surgery, unless it is needed because of accidental injury or to improve the function of a malformed part of the body, (6) most prescription drugs, (7) custodial care at home or in a nursing home and (8) orthopedic shoes.

Charges imposed by an immediate relative (e.g., a doctor who is the son/daughter or brother/sister of the patient) are *not* covered.

Doctors cannot make self-referrals for certain designated health services. Designated health services include any of the following items or services: (1) clinical laboratory services, (2) physical therapy services, (3) occupational therapy services, (4) radiology services, including MRI, CAT scans, and ultrasound services, (5) radiation therapy services and supplies, (6) durable medical equipment and supplies, (7) parenteral and enteral nutrients, equipment, and supplies, (8) prosthetics, orthotics, and prosthetic devices and supplies, (9) home health services, (10) outpatient prescription drugs, and (11) inpatient and outpatient hospital services.

The law prohibits a doctor who has a financial relationship with an entity from referring Medicare patients to that entity to receive a designated health service. The prohibition also applies if a doctor's immediate family member has a financial relationship with an entity. A financial relationship can exist as an ownership or investment interest in or a compensation arrangement with an entity. The law is triggered by the mere fact that a financial relationship exists; it does not matter what the doctor intends when making a referral. An entity cannot bill Medicare, Medicaid, the beneficiary, or anyone else for a designated health service furnished to a Medicare patient under a prohibited referral.

The law prohibits Medicare payments for designated health services in violation of the law. If a person collects any amount for services billed in violation of the law, a refund must be made. A person can be subject to a civil money penalty or exclusion from Medicare if that person (1) presents or causes to be presented a claim to Medicare or bill to any individual, third party payer, or other entity for any designated health service the person knows or should know was furnished as a result of a prohibited referral, or (2) fails to make a timely refund.

C-17. What outpatient hospital services are covered under Medical Insurance?

Medical Insurance (Part B) helps pay for covered services a patient receives as an outpatient from a participating hospital for diagnosis or treatment of an illness or injury. Under certain conditions, Medical Insurance helps pay for emergency outpatient care the patient receives from a non-participating hospital. The patient must meet the annual Medical Insurance deductible before Medicare will begin paying for outpatient hospital charges and then pay a 20% copayment.

Major outpatient hospital services covered by Medical Insurance include (1) services in an emergency room or outpatient clinic, including same-day surgery, (2) laboratory tests billed by the hospital, (3) mental health care in a partial hospitalization psychiatric program, if a physician certifies that inpatient treatment would be required without it, (4) X-rays and other radiology services billed by the hospital, (5) medical supplies such as splints and casts, (6) drugs and biologicals that cannot be self-administered, and (7) blood transfusions furnished to the patient as an outpatient (after the first three pints).

Outpatient hospital services not covered by Medical Insurance include (1) most routine physical examinations and tests directly related to the examinations, (2) eye or ear examinations to prescribe or fit eyeglasses or hearing aids, (3) most immunizations, (4) most prescription drugs, (5) most routine foot care and (6) most dental care.

C-18. When are outpatient physical therapy and speech-language pathology services covered?

Outpatient physical therapy and speech-language pathology services are covered if received as part of a patient's treatment in a doctor's office or as an outpatient of a participating hospital, skilled nursing facility, or home health agency; or approved clinic, rehabilitative agency, or public health agency. Services must be furnished under a plan established by a physician or physical therapist. A physician is required to review all plans of care.

A podiatrist (when acting within the scope of his practice) is a physician for purposes of establishing a plan for outpatient physical therapy. A dentist and podiatrist are also within the definition of a physician for purposes of outpatient ambulatory surgery in a physician's office.

Separate calendar year caps ($1,780 in 2007) on coverage of independent occupational therapy and physical and speech therapy services returned January 1, 2006. The annual limitation was initially enacted for 1999, but Congress granted and then extended a moratorium on implementation through the end of 2002. Implementation was further delayed by administration decision until September 1, 2003. The limitation was then eliminated effective December 7, 2003. The Medicare Prescription Drug, Improvement, and Modernization Act of 2003 eliminated the annual limit through the end of 2005. In the Deficit Reduction Act of 2005, Congress added a provision for the Secretary of Health and Human Services to make an exception to the annual limit if the provision of additional services is "medically necessary." The exceptions process allows for specific diagnoses and procedures to receive Medicare coverage even after a beneficiary has met their therapy cap for the year. Alternatively, a provider can request an exception if the particular problem to be treated is not automatically covered under the given exceptions. This exceptions process was scheduled to end January 1, 2007, but has been extended through December 31, 2007.

When effective, the limit applies to all outpatient physical therapy services (including speech-language pathology services) except for services furnished by a hospital outpatient department. A separate limit also applies to all outpatient occupational therapy services except for services furnished by hospital outpatient departments. Therapy services furnished incident to a physician's professional services are also subject to the limits.

C-19. Are partial hospitalization services incident to physician's services covered?

Yes. Partial hospitalization services (sometimes called day treatments) are items and services prescribed by a physician and provided in a program under the supervision of a physician pursuant to an individualized written plan of treatment.

The program must be furnished by a hospital to its outpatients or by a community mental health center and must be in a distinct and organized intensive ambulatory treatment service offering less than 24 hour daily care.

Covered items and services include the following:

- individual and group therapy with physicians or psychologists (or other mental health professionals to the extent authorized by state law),

- occupational therapy requiring the skills of a qualified occupational therapist,

- services of social workers, trained psychiatric nurses, and other staff trained to work with psychiatric patients,

- drugs and biologicals furnished for therapeutic purposes (which cannot be self-administered),

- individualized activity therapies that are not primarily recreational or diversionary,

- family counseling (the primary purpose of which is treatment of the individual's condition),

- patient training and education (to the extent that training and educational activities are closely and clearly related to the individual's care and treatment),

- diagnostic services, and

- other necessary items and services (not including meals and transportation).

C-20. Are certified nurse-midwife services covered under Medical Insurance?

Yes. A certified nurse-midwife is a registered professional nurse who meets the following requirements:

(1) is currently licensed to practice in the state as a nurse-midwife in the state where services are performed,

(2) has completed a program of study and clinical experience for nurse-midwives that is accredited by an accrediting body approved by the U.S. Department of Education, and

(3) is certified as a nurse-midwife by the American College of Nurse-Midwives or the American College of Nurse-Midwives Certification Council.

Certified nurse-midwife services are services furnished by a certified nurse-midwife and such services and supplies as are incident to nurse-midwife service. The service must be authorized under state law.

The definition of nurse-midwife services includes coverage of services outside the maternity cycle.

The amount paid by Medical Insurance for such services is based upon a fee schedule but cannot exceed 65% of the prevailing charge allowed for the same service performed by a physician.

C-21. Is dental work covered under Medical Insurance?

Medical Insurance helps pay for services of a dentist in certain cases when the medical problem is more extensive than the teeth or structures directly supporting the teeth. Dental work for jaw or facial bone surgery, whether required because of accident or disease, is covered. If a patient needs to be hospitalized because of the severity of a dental procedure, Hospital Insurance may pay for the patient's inpatient hospital stay even if the dental care itself is not covered by Medicare.

Medical Insurance generally does not pay for routine dental care such as the treatment, filling, removal, or replacement of teeth; root canal therapy; surgery for impacted teeth; or other surgical procedures involving the teeth or structures directly supporting the teeth.

C-22. What medical equipment is covered under Medical Insurance?

The following medical equipment is covered: surgical dressings, splints, casts and other devices for reduction of fractures and dislocations; rental or purchase of durable medical equipment, such as iron lungs, oxygen tents, hospital beds and wheelchairs, for use in the patient's home; prosthetic devices, such as artificial heart valves or synthetic arteries, designed to replace part or all of an internal organ (but not false teeth, hearing aids, or eyeglasses); colostomy or ileostomy bags and certain related supplies; breast prostheses (including a surgical brassiere) after a mastectomy; braces for arm, leg, back, or neck; and artificial limbs and eyes. Orthopedic shoes are not covered unless they are part of leg braces and the cost is included in the orthopedist's charge. Adhesive tape, antiseptics, and other common first-aid supplies are also not included.

Durable medical equipment is equipment that must be able to be used over again by other patients, must primarily serve a medical purpose, must not be useful to people who are not sick or injured, and must be appropriate for use in the patient's home. Medical Insurance pays for different kinds of durable medical equipment in different ways; some equipment must be rented, other equipment must be purchased, and for some equipment the patient may choose rental or purchase. A doctor should prescribe medical equipment for the patient.

Suppliers of medical equipment and supplies (durable medical equipment, prosthetic devices, orthotics and prosthetics, surgical dressings, home dialysis supplies and equipment, immunosuppressive drugs, therapeutic shoes for diabetics, oral cancer drugs, and self-administered erythropoietin) are not reimbursed by Medicare for these items unless they have a Medicare supplier number. A supplier cannot obtain a supplier number unless the supplier meets uniform national standards.

The standards require suppliers to (1) comply with all applicable state and federal licensure and regulatory requirements, (2) maintain a physical facility, (3) have proof of appropriate liability insurance, and (4) meet other requirements established by the Centers for Medicare & Medicaid Services. The requirement for suppliers to obtain a supplier number does not apply to medical equipment and supplies furnished as incident to a physician's service.

C-23. Is ambulance service covered by Medical Insurance?

Yes, Medical Insurance helps pay for the "reasonable costs" of medically necessary ambulance transportation, including air ambulance, but only if the patient's condition does not permit the use of other methods of transportation and the ambulance, equipment and personnel meet Medicare requirements. Medical Insurance can help pay for ambulance transportation from the scene of an accident to a hospital, from a patient's home to a hospital or skilled nursing facility, between hospitals and skilled nursing facilities, or from a hospital or skilled nursing facility to the patient's home. Also, if the patient is an inpatient in a hospital or skilled nursing facility which cannot provide a medically necessary service, Medical Insurance can help pay for round trip ambulance transportation to the nearest appropriate facility. Medicare does not pay for ambulance use from a patient's home to a doctor's office.

Medicare also does not pay for ambulance use from the patient's home to a dialysis facility that is not in or next to a hospital.

Medical Insurance usually can help pay for ambulance transportation only in the patient's local area. But if there are no local facilities equipped to provide the care the patient needs, Medical Insurance helps pay for necessary ambulance transportation to the closest facility outside the patient's local area that can provide the necessary care. If the patient chooses to go to another institution that is farther away, Medicare payment will be based on the reasonable charge for transportation to the closest facility.

Necessary ambulance services in connection with a covered inpatient stay in a Canadian or Mexican hospital can also be covered by Medical Insurance.

Medicare pays for use of an air ambulance only in extremely urgent emergency situations. If a patient could have been moved by land ambulance without serious danger to life or health, Medicare pays only the land ambulance rate. The patient is responsible for the difference between the air ambulance rate and the land ambulance rate.

C-24. How much will Medicare pay for outpatient treatment of mental illness?

Medical Insurance helps pay the cost of outpatient mental health services a patient receives from physicians, clinical psychologists, clinical social workers and other nonphysician practitioners. When treatment is furnished on an outpatient basis, mental health treatment services are subject to a payment limitation that is called "outpatient mental health limitation." In effect, once the annual deductible is met, Medical Insurance pays only 50% (not 80%) of the approved amount for these services. In other words, the patient is responsible for paying 50% coinsurance instead of the usual 20% for these services. On assigned claims, beneficiaries are responsible for paying 50% of the approved amount. For unassigned claims, beneficiaries may have to pay more.

Partial hospitalization services (except those furnished by a physician) for treatment of mental illness are not subject to this payment limitation. Also, brief office visits for the sole purpose of monitoring or changing drug prescriptions used in the treatment of mental illness are not subject to this payment limitation.

Partial hospitalization (sometimes called day treatment) is a program of outpatient mental health care. Partial hospitalization services mean a distinct and organized intensive ambulatory treatment program that offers less than 24-hour daily care and furnishes mental health care services. Under certain conditions, Medical Insurance helps pay for these programs when provided by hospital outpatient departments or by community mental health centers.

The Centers for Medicare & Medicaid Services defines community mental health centers as any entity that (1) provides outpatient services, including specialized out-patient services for children, the elderly, individuals who are chronically mentally ill, and residents of its mental health service area who have been discharged from inpatient treatment at a mental health facility; (2) provides 24-hour-a-day emergency care services; (3) provides day treatment or other partial hospitalization services, or psychosocial reha-bilitation services; (4) provides screening for patients being considered for admission to state mental health facilities; (5) provides consultation and education services; and (6) meets applicable licensing or certification requirements for community mental health centers in the state in which it is located.

C-25. When is the cost of vaccines covered?

The cost of pneumonia pneumococcal vaccine is covered, and the cost of hepatitis B vaccine for high and intermediate risk individuals is covered when it is administered in a hospital or renal dialysis facility. Also covered is the cost of flu vaccine and its administration. Neither the annual deductible nor the 20% coinsurance applies to flu and pneumonia vaccines. If the person giving the patient the shot accepts assignment (accepts the Medicare payment as payment in full), there will be no cost to the patient. If the person does not accept assignment, the patient may have to pay charges in ad-dition to the Medicare approved amount. A patient must have doctor's orders to get a pneumonia shot. Any health care professional complying with the Medicare rules can give a patient a flu shot.

C-26. Is the cost of antigens covered?

Under certain circumstances, Medical Insurance helps pay for antigens prepared for the patient by a doctor. A patient should check with the area Medicare carrier to determine if Medical Insurance will pay for the antigens.

C-27. When is a liver transplant covered under Medical Insurance?

The Department of Health and Human Services is implementing a policy under which a liver transplant is not considered an experimental procedure for Medicare beneficiaries solely because an individual is over 18 years of age.

A liver transplant will be covered when reasonably and medically necessary. The Department of Health and Human Services will place appropriate limiting criteria on coverage, disease state, and the institution providing the care, so as to ensure the highest quality of medical care demonstrated to be consistent with successful outcomes.

C-28. Can Medical Insurance help pay for outpatient services at a comprehensive outpatient rehabilitation facility?

Under certain circumstances, Medical Insurance helps pay for outpatient services re-ceived from a Medicare-participating comprehensive outpatient rehabilitation facility

(CORF). Outpatient services must be performed by a doctor or other qualified professional. Covered services include physicians' services; physical, speech, occupation and respiratory therapies; counseling; and other related services. A patient must be referred by a physician who certifies that there is a need for skilled rehabilitation services. For most CORF services, the patient is responsible only for the annual deductible and 20% of the Medicare approved-charges. Medicare also helps pay for mental health treatment in a CORF.

C-29. Are home health services covered under Medical Insurance?

In a process that began in 1998, home health services not directly related to hospital or skilled nursing facility stays are now covered and paid for by Medical Insurance (Part B). These services tend to be for chronic conditions, and are different from home care services needed for convalescence and rehabilitation following a hospital stay. Medicare pays for the costs of part-time skilled care (no co-pay) and 80% of the cost of durable medical equipment when suppled by a certified home health agency. The trust fund transfer for this benefit was phased in over a six-year period, while the cost of the home health services transferred was phased in to the Part B premium over seven years.

C-30. Are independent clinical laboratory services covered?

All laboratories must be certified under the Clinical Laboratory Improvement Amendments to perform laboratory testing. Medical Insurance pays the full approved fee for covered clinical diagnostic tests provided by certified laboratories that are participating in Medicare. The laboratory can be independent, part of a hospital outpatient department, or in a doctor's office. The laboratory must accept assignment for the tests. It may not bill the patient for the tests.

C-31. Are screening pap smears and pelvic exams covered?

Generally, a screening pap smear and pelvic exam (including a clinical breast exam) are covered every two years. Annual coverage is provided for women (1) at high risk for cervical or vaginal cancer, or (2) of childbearing age who have had a pap smear during the preceding three years indicating the presence of cervical or vaginal cancer or other abnormality. The Part B deductible is waived for screening pap smears and pelvic exams. Pelvic exams are paid under the physician fee schedule.

C-32. Are breast cancer screening and diagnostic mammography covered?

Screening and diagnostic mammography are covered. "Screening mammography" is defined as a radiologic procedure furnished to a woman without signs or symptoms of breast disease, for the purpose of early detection of breast cancer, and includes a physician's interpretation of the results of the procedure. "Diagnostic mammography" means a radiologic procedure furnished to a man or woman with signs or symptoms of breast disease, or a personal history of breast cancer, or a personal history of biopsy-proven benign breast disease, and includes a physicians's interpretation of the results of the procedure. Medicare covers an annual screening mammogram for all women age 40 and over. The Part B deductible for screening mammography is waived.

C-33. Are prostate screening tests covered under Part B?

Annual prostate cancer screening for men age 50 and older is covered. Covered procedures include (1) digital rectal exam, (2) prostate-specific antigen (PSA) blood test, and (3) other procedures that the Department of Health and Human Services finds appropriate. Payment for the PSA blood test will be made under the clinical laboratory fee schedule, and other services will be paid under the physician fee schedule.

C-34. How is colorectal screening covered?

Covered colorectal screening procedures include (1) an annual fecal occult blood test for persons age 50 and over, (2) flexible sigmoidoscopy for persons age 50 and over to be done once every four years, and (3) colonoscopy for persons at high risk for colorectal cancer once every two years. The physician may substitute a barium enema for a sigmoidoscopy or colonoscopy in his discretion.

C-35. Are diabetes self-management benefits covered?

Services furnished in non-hospital-based programs for diabetes outpatient self-management training are covered. (Services furnished in hospital-based programs were already covered.) Services may be provided by physicians or other entities designated by the Department of Health and Human Services if they also provide other services paid by Medicare and meet quality standards. A physician managing the patient's condition must certify that the services are needed under a comprehensive plan of care.

Coverage includes blood glucose monitors and testing strips for all diabetics (already covered for insulin-dependent diabetics), lancets and self-management training. Medicare also covers medical nutrition therapy services provided by a dietitian or nutrition professional. Since 2005, coverage includes diabetes screening tests for those at risk of getting diabetes.

C-36. When does Medicare cover bone mass measurements?

Medical Insurance (Part B) covers procedures to identify bone mass, detect bone loss, or determine bone quality, including a physician's interpretation of the results. Persons qualifying for these procedures include estrogen-deficient women at risk for osteoporosis, and persons: (1) with vertebral abnormalities, (2) receiving long-term glucocorticoid steroid therapy, (3) with primary hyperparathyroidism, and (4) being monitored to assess the response to, or efficacy of, an approved osteoporosis drug.

C-37. Under what conditions is an injectable drug for post-menopausal osteoporosis covered?

The cost of an injectable drug for the treatment of a bone fracture related to post-menopausal osteoporosis is covered under the following conditions: (1) the patient's attending physician certifies that the patient is unable to learn the skills needed to self-administer (or is physically or mentally incapable of administering) the drug, and (2) the patient meets the requirements for Medicare coverage of home health services.

C-38. When are eyeglasses covered under Medicare?

Medical Insurance will pay for one pair of conventional eyeglasses or conventional contact lenses if necessary after cataract surgery with insertion of an intraocular lens.

Medical Insurance will pay for cataract spectacles, cataract contact lenses, or intraocular lenses that replace the natural lens of the eye after cataract surgery. Medical Insurance will not pay for routine eye exams and usually will not pay for eyeglasses.

C-39. Under what circumstances are the services of nurse practitioners and clinical nurse specialists in rural areas covered?

The services of nurse practitioners and clinical nurse specialists are covered when the services performed are those authorized under state law and regulations, provided there is no facility or other provider charges paid in connection with the service. Also, a clinical nurse specialist must be a registered nurse licensed to practice in the state who holds a Master's degree in a defined clinical area of nursing and from an accredited educational institution.

C-40. When are lung and heart-lung transplants covered under Medical Insurance?

Medicare covers lung transplants for beneficiaries with progressive end-stage pulmonary disease when performed by facilities that (1) make an application to the Centers for Medicare & Medicaid Services for approval as a lung transplant facility, (2) supply documentation showing their satisfaction of compliance with federal regulations on lung transplants, and (3) are approved by the Centers for Medicare & Medicaid Services under criteria based on federal regulations. Medicare also covers lung transplantation for end-stage cardiopulmonary disease when it is expected that transplant of the lung will result in improved cardiac function.

In addition, Medicare covers heart-lung transplants for beneficiaries with progressive end-stage cardiopulmonary disease when they are provided in a facility that has been approved by Medicare for both heart and lung transplantation.

Facilities must meet specific criteria in areas such as patient selection, patient management, commitment, plans, experience and survival rates, maintenance of data, organ procurement, laboratory services, and billing. Facilities must have patient selection criteria for determining suitable candidates for lung transplants.

For facilities that are approved to perform lung transplants, Medicare covers under Hospital Insurance (Part A) all medically reasonable and necessary inpatient services. (See Section B for discussion of Hospital Insurance.) Physician services, as well as other non-hospital services related to the transplant, and pre- and post-transplant care, may be covered under Medical Insurance (Part B) and paid under the physician fee schedule or on a reasonable cost basis or other basis. Under certain circumstances, kidney and liver transplants also may be covered.

C-41. Are prescription drugs used in immunosuppressive therapy covered under Medical Insurance?

Payment may be made for prescription drugs used in immunosuppressive therapy that have been approved for marketing by the Food and Drug Administration and that meet one of the following conditions:

(1) The approved labeling includes the indication for preventing or treating the rejection of a transplanted organ or tissue.

(2) The approved labeling includes the indication for use in conjunction with immunosuppressive drugs to prevent or treat rejection of a transplanted organ or tissue.

(3) The drugs have been determined by a carrier, in processing a Medicare claim, to be reasonable and necessary for the specific purpose of preventing or treating the rejection of a patient's transplanted organ or tissue, or for use in conjunction with immunosuppressive drugs for the purpose of preventing or treating the rejection of a patient's transplanted organ or tissue.

Coverage under Medical Insurance is available only for prescription drugs used in immunosuppressive therapy, furnished to an individual who receives an organ or tissue transplant for which Medicare payment is made, for up to 36 months after the date of discharge from the hospital during which the covered transplant was performed.

Drugs are covered irrespective of whether they can be self-administered.

C-42. Are ambulatory surgical services covered under Medical Insurance (Part B)?

An ambulatory surgical center is a facility that provides surgical services that do not require a hospital stay. Medical Insurance will pay for the use of an ambulatory surgical center for certain approved surgical procedures. The center must have an agreement to participate in the Medicare program. Medicare also helps pay for physician and anesthesia services that are provided in connection with the procedure.

C-43. When are rural health clinic services covered by Medical Insurance?

Medical Insurance helps pay for services of physicians, nurse practitioners, physician assistants, nurse midwives, visiting nurses (under certain circumstances), clinical psychologists, and clinical social workers furnished by a rural health clinic. Medical Insurance also helps pay for certain laboratory tests in these clinics. The patient is responsible for the annual Medical Insurance deductible plus 20% of the Medicare-approved charge for the clinic.

Rural health clinics must meet requirements concerning where they are located. They must be in areas where there are insufficient numbers of needed health care practitioners (not just primary care physicians). Clinics that no longer meet the shortage area requirements will be permitted to retain their designation only if the Department of Health and Human Services determines that they are essential to the delivery of primary care services that would otherwise be unavailable in the area.

C-44. Is there Medicare reimbursement for telehealth services in rural areas?

Part B payments are made for professional consultation via telecommunications systems with a health care provider furnishing a service for which Medicare payment would be made for a beneficiary residing in a rural county that was designated as a health professional shortage area. In determining the amount of payments for telehealth services, the payments are subject to Medicare coinsurance and deductible requirements, and balanced billing applies to services furnished by non-participating physicians. Beneficiaries are not to be billed for any telephone line charges or any facility fees. In addition, payment for telehealth services are increased annually by the update factor for physicians' services under the fee schedule.

C-45. Does Medical Insurance help pay for federally qualified health center services?

Federally qualified health centers are located in both rural and urban areas and any Medicare beneficiary may seek services at them. As part of the "federally qualified health center benefit," Medical Insurance helps pay for the following outpatient services:

(1) physician services,

(2) services and supplies furnished as incident to a physician's professional services,

(3) nurse practitioner or physician assistant services,

(4) services and supplies furnished as incident to a nurse practitioner or physician assistant services,

(5) clinical psychologist and clinical social worker services,

(6) services and supplies furnished as incident to a clinical psychologist or clinical social worker services,

(7) visiting nurse services,

(8) nurse-midwife services, and

(9) preventive primary services.

Preventive primary services include medical social services, nutritional assessment and referral, preventive health education, children's eye and ear examinations, prenatal and post-partum screening, immunizations, voluntary family planning services, and services outlined in the recommendations of the U.S. Preventive Services Task Force for patients age 65 and older. Preventive services do not include eyeglasses, hearing aids, group or mass information programs or health education classes, or preventive dental services. Preventive services covered under special provisions of Medicare, such as screening mammography, may be provided by a federally qualified health center only if the center meets the special provisions that govern those benefits.

The patient does not have to pay the Medical Insurance annual deductible for services provided under the federally qualified health center benefit. The patient is responsible for 20% of the Medicare-approved charge for the clinic. Federally qualified health centers often provide services in addition to those offered under the Medicare federally qualified health center benefit. Examples of these services are X-rays and equipment like crutches and canes. As long as the center meets Medicare requirements to provide these services, Medical Insurance can help pay for them. The patient is responsible for any unmet part of the annual Medical Insurance deductible plus 20% of the Medicare-approved charge for the service.

C-46. What other benefits are provided under Medical Insurance?

Additional benefits include the following:

- The cost of *blood clotting factors and supplies* related to their administration for hemophilia patients who are able to use them to control bleeding without medical or other supervision. The amount of clotting factors necessary to have on hand for a specific period is determined for each patient individually.

- *Outpatient radiation therapy* given under the supervision of a doctor.

- *Oral anti-nausea drugs used as part of an anti-cancer chemotherapeutic regimen.* The drug must be administered by a physician (or prescribed by a physician) for use immediately before, at, or within 48 hours after the time of administration of the chemotherapeutic agent and used as a full replacement for the anti-emetic therapy which would otherwise be administered intravenously.

- *Portable diagnostic X-ray services* received by a patient at home or at other locations if they are ordered by a doctor and if they are provided by a Medicare-approved supplier.

- Under certain circumstances, *liver and kidney transplants* in a Medicare-approved facility.

- *Prosthetic devices* needed to replace an internal body organ. These include Medicare-approved corrective lenses needed after a cataract operation, ostomy bags and certain related supplies, and breast prostheses (including a surgical brassiere) after a mastectomy. Medical Insurance also helps pay for artificial limbs and eyes, and for arm, leg, back, and neck braces. Medical Insurance does not pay for orthopedic shoes unless they are an integral part of leg braces and the cost is included in the charge for the braces. Medical Insurance does not pay for dental plates or other dental devices.

- The drug *Epoetin alfa* when used to treat Medicare beneficiaries with anemia related to chronic kidney failure, or related to use of AZT in HIV-positive beneficiaries or for other uses that a Medicare carrier finds medically appropriate. The Epoetin alfa must be administered incident to the services of a doctor in the office or in a hospital outpatient department. Medical Insurance also helps pay for Epoetin alfa that is self-administered by home dialysis patients or administered by their caregivers.

- *Oral cancer drugs* if they are the same chemical entity as those administered intravenously and covered prior to 1994. In addition, off-label anti-cancer drugs are covered in some cases.

C-47. What services are covered with no cost sharing?

A patient does not have to pay the annual deductible or the 20% coinsurance for the following services: (1) the cost of second opinions for certain surgical procedures when Medicare requires a second opinion, (2) the cost of home health services except the 20% coinsurance charge applies for durable medical equipment (except for the purchase of certain used items), (3) flu shot and pneumococcal vaccine, and (4) outpatient clinical diagnostic laboratory tests performed by physicians who take assignments, or by hospitals or independent laboratories that are Medicare-certified.

MEDICARE COVERAGE OF BLOOD

C-48. Does Medicare help pay for blood?

Both Hospital Insurance and Medical Insurance can help pay for blood (whole blood or units of packed red blood cells), blood components, and the cost of blood processing and administration.

If a patient receives blood as an inpatient of a hospital or skilled nursing facility, Hospital Insurance will pay all of the blood costs, except for a deductible charged for the first three pints of whole blood or units of packed red cells in each benefit period. The deductible is the charge that some hospitals and skilled nursing facilities make for blood which is not replaced.

The patient is responsible for the deductible for the first three pints or units of blood furnished by a hospital or skilled nursing facility in a calendar year. If the patient is charged a deductible, he has the option of either paying the deductible or having the blood replaced. A hospital or skilled nursing facility cannot charge a patient for any of the first three pints of blood he replaces. Any blood deductible satisfied under Medical Insurance will reduce the blood deductible requirements under Hospital Insurance.

Medical Insurance can help pay for blood and blood components received as an out-patient or as part of other covered services, except for a deductible charged for the first three pints or units received in each calendar year. After the patient has met the annual deductible, Medical Insurance pays 80% of the approved charge for blood starting with the fourth pint in a calendar year.

PRIVATE CONTRACTS

C-49. Can physicians enter into private contracts with Medicare beneficiaries?

Yes, physicians or practitioners can sign private contracts with Medicare beneficiaries for which no claim is to be submitted to Medicare and for which the physician or practitioner receives no reimbursement from Medicare, on a capitated basis, or from an organization that receives reimbursement under Medicare for the item or service. Services provided under private contracts are not covered under Medicare.

A private contract is not valid unless it (1) is written and signed by the beneficiary before any item or service is provided pursuant to the contract, (2) is entered into when the beneficiary is not facing an emergency or urgent health care situation, and (3) contains specific items listed below.

Among other provisions, the contract must clearly indicate to the beneficiary that by signing the contract the beneficiary (1) agrees not to submit a claim to Medicare even if the items or services would otherwise by covered, (2) agrees to be responsible, through insurance or otherwise, for payment of the items and services and understands that no reimbursement will be provided under Medicare, (3) acknowledges that no limits will apply to amounts that could be charged for the items and services, (4) acknowledges that Medigap plans do not make payments for these items and services because Medicare does not make payment, and (5) acknowledges that the beneficiary has a right to have the items and services provided by other physicians or practitioners for whom payment would be made under Medicare.

Private contracts are not valid unless the physician files an affidavit with the Department of Health and Human Services not later than 10 days after the first contract to which the affidavit applies is entered into. The affidavit must identify the physician or practitioner, be signed by the physician or practitioner, and provide that, except for emergency services, the physician or practitioner will not submit any claim to Medicare for any item or service provided to *any* beneficiary for two years beginning on the date the affidavit is signed.

If the physician or practitioner knowingly and willfully submits a claim to Medicare for any item or service furnished to a beneficiary (except emergency services) during the two-year period, (1) the physician or practitioner will no longer be allowed to furnish services under private contracts for the remainder of the two-year period, and (2) no Medicare payment will be made for any item or service furnished by the physician or practitioner during the remainder of the two year period.

PART C:
MEDICARE ADVANTAGE

DEFINITION

D-1. What is Medicare Advantage?

Medicare Advantage (formerly known as Medicare+Choice) permits contracts between the Centers for Medicare & Medicaid Services and a variety of different managed care and fee-for-service entities. Most Medicare beneficiaries may choose to receive benefits through the original Medicare fee-for-service program or through one of the following Medicare Advantage plans:

- Coordinated care plans, including Health Maintenance Organizations (HMOs), Preferred Provider Organizations (PPOs), and Provider-Sponsored Organizations (PSOs).

- Private fee-for-service plans which reimburse providers on a fee-for-service basis, and are authorized to charge enrolled beneficiaries up to 115% of the plan's payment schedule (which may be different from the Medicare fee schedule).

Since 2005, Medicare Advantage provides for regional preferred provider plans. These plans benefit from unique financial and administrative provisions and incentives under the Medicare Prescription Drug, Improvement, and Modernization Act of 2003.

D-2. What is a health maintenance organization (HMO)?

An HMO is a managed care plan that provides to its members, who are also Medicare beneficiaries, either directly or through arrangement with others, at least all the Medicare covered services that are available to Medicare beneficiaries who are not enrolled in the HMO who reside in the geographic area serviced by the HMO. Some HMOs also provide services not covered by Medicare, either free to the Medicare enrollee (that is, funded out of the payment Medicare makes to the HMO) or for an additional charge. HMOs typically charge a set monthly premium and nominal copayments for services instead of Medicare's coinsurance and deductibles.

Each plan has its own network of hospitals, skilled nursing facilities, home health agencies, doctors, and other professionals. Depending on how the plan is organized, services are usually provided either at one or more centrally located health facilities or in the private practice offices of the doctors and other health care professionals that are part of the plan. A beneficiary generally must receive all covered care through the plan or from health care professionals referred to by the plan.

Most managed health plans allow the beneficiary to select a primary care doctor from those that are part of the plan. If the beneficiary does not make a selection, one will be assigned. The primary care doctor is responsible for managing the beneficiaries' medical care, including admitting the beneficiary to a hospital or referring the beneficiary

71

to specialists. The beneficiary is allowed to change the primary care doctor as long as another primary care doctor affiliated with the plan is selected.

Before enrolling in a managed care plan, the beneficiary should find out whether the plan has a "risk" or a "cost" contract with Medicare. There is an important difference.

Risk Plans. These plans have "lock-in" requirements. This means that the beneficiary generally is locked into receiving all covered care through the plan or through referrals by the plan. In most cases, if the beneficiary receives services that are not authorized by the plan, neither the plan nor Medicare will pay. The only exceptions recognized by all Medicare-contracting plans are for emergency services, which the beneficiary may receive anywhere in the United States, and for services the beneficiary urgently needs when temporarily out of the plan's service area.

Cost Plans. These plans do not have lock-in requirements. If a beneficiary enrolls in a cost plan, he can either go to health care providers affiliated with the plan or go outside the plan. If a beneficiary goes outside the plan, the plan probably will not pay but Medicare will. Medicare will pay its share of charges it approves. The beneficiary will be responsible for Medicare's coinsurance, deductibles, and other charges, just as if receiving care under the regular Medicare program.

D-3. What is a Medicare Advantage private fee-for-service plan?

A private fee-for-service plan is defined as a plan that reimburses doctors, hospitals and other providers on a fee-for-service basis, does not place them at risk, does not vary payment rates based on utilization, and does not restrict which doctor or hospital the member can use. The insurance plan, rather than the Medicare program, decides how much to reimburse for services received by the beneficiary. The beneficiary pays the Part B premium ($93.50 in 2007 for most beneficiaries), any monthly premium the private fee-for-service plan charges, and an amount per visit or service.

D-4. What is a Provider-Sponsored Organization (PSO)?

PSOs are public or private entities established by or organized by a health care provider, such as a hospital, or a group of affiliated health care providers, such as a geriatric unit of a hospital, that provide a substantial proportion of health care items and services directly through that provider or group. Affiliated providers share, directly or indirectly, substantial financial risk and have at least a majority financial interest in the PSO.

D-5. What is a religious fraternal benefit society plan?

These plans may restrict enrollment to members of the church, convention, or group with which the society is affiliated. They must meet Medicare financial solvency requirements and Medicare may adjust payment amounts to these plans to take into account the actuarial characteristics and experience of plan enrollees.

ELIGIBILITY, ELECTION, AND ENROLLMENT

D-6. What is the enrollment/disenrollment process for Medicare Advantage?

Beneficiaries entitled to Hospital Insurance (Part A) and enrolled in Medical Insurance (Part B) are eligible to enroll in a plan that serves the geographic area in which they reside, except beneficiaries with end-stage renal disease (although beneficiaries who develop end-stage renal disease may remain in the plan if already enrolled) and beneficiaries receiving inpatient hospice care. Part B only enrollees are ineligible.

The Centers for Medicare & Medicaid Services has established procedures for enrollment and disenrollment in Medicare Advantage options. Newly eligible enrollees who do not choose a Medicare Advantage plan are deemed to have chosen the original Medicare fee-for-service option, except that the Centers for Medicare & Medicaid Services may (but has not done so) establish procedures under which "age-ins" enrolled in a plan with a Medicare Advantage contract are deemed to have elected that plan for their Medicare coverage. Individuals remain enrolled in the option of their choice until they choose another plan.

D-7. What are the enrollment periods?

Beneficiaries can choose a Medicare Advantage plan at initial eligibility or during one of the enrollment periods described below. From 1998 through 2004, they could enroll (if the plan was open to new enrollees) or disenroll on a monthly basis. For the first six months of 2005 (or the first six months of eligibility in year 2005, in the case of person first eligible for Medicare Advantage in 2005), beneficiaries could enroll and disenroll from plans, but they could only change plans once during that period. The same process applies in years after 2005, except that the freedom to change must be done in the first three months of the year (or the first three months of eligibility) or during the annual coordinated enrollment period:

- The annual coordinated enrollment period runs from November 15 through December 31 of each year. Enrollments at this time are effective the following January 1. In conjunction with the annual coordinated enrollment period, the Department of Health and Human Services must sponsor a "Health Information Fair" to publicize Medicare Advantage options.

- Beginning in 2002, special election periods are available in which a beneficiary can disenroll if the plan was terminated, the beneficiary moved out of the plan's service area, the beneficiary demonstrates that the plan violated its contract or misrepresented the plan in marketing, or any other conditions specified by the Centers for Medicare & Medicaid Services.

- Also, beginning in 2002, newly eligible beneficiaries who elect a Medicare Advantage option may disenroll into the original Medicare fee-for-service option any time during the first 12 months of their enrollment.

Plans must accept all beneficiaries on a first-come-first-serve basis, subject to capacity limits.

Plans may only disenroll beneficiaries for cause (i.e., failure to pay premiums or disruptive behavior) or plan termination in the beneficiary's geographic area. Beneficiaries terminated for cause are enrolled in the original Medicare fee-for-service program. Others may have a special election period.

Medicare Advantage plans must submit marketing materials, including application forms, to the Centers for Medicare & Medicaid Services at least 45 days prior to distribution. The material must be approved by the Department of Health and Human Services. Medicare Advantage plans must conform to fair marketing standards, including a prohibition on the plan from offering cash or rebates. If a plan's marketing materials were approved for one service area, they will be deemed to be approved in all of the plan's service areas, except in regard to area-specific information.

Note: Organizations cannot contract to enroll Medicare beneficiaries under the Medicare Advantage program until they have met standards of the Department of Health and Human Services.

D-8. How is information provided to beneficiaries?

At least 15 days before the required November coordinated election period (see D-7), the Centers for Medicare & Medicaid Services must mail to each beneficiary general information on Medicare and comparative information on Medicare Advantage plans available in their area. General information includes information on covered benefits, cost sharing, and balance billing liability under the original fee-for-service program; election procedures; grievance and appeals rights; and information on Medigap insurance and Medicare SELECT. Comparative information includes extensive information on benefits and beneficiary liability; premiums; service areas; quality and performance; and supplemental benefits. The Centers for Medicare & Medicaid Services must make available a toll-free number for inquiries on Medicare Advantage options and an Internet site providing information on Medicare Advantage options.

BENEFITS AND BENEFICIARY PROTECTIONS

D-9. What basic benefits are provided by Medicare Advantage plans?

All Medicare Advantage plans are required to provide the current Medicare benefit package (excluding hospice services) and any additional health services required under the adjusted community rate (ACR) process.

Medicare Advantage plans may offer mandatory supplemental benefits, subject to approval by the Centers for Medicare & Medicaid Services. Mandatory supplemental benefits must be approved unless it is determined that offering such benefits would substantially discourage enrollment. Medicare Advantage plans may also offer optional supplemental benefits. Private fee-for-service plans may offer supplemental benefits that include payment for some or all of the permitted balance billings amounts and additional services that the plan determines are medically necessary.

Medicare Advantage plans must provide payments to non-contracting providers or other persons so that the total payments (the plan's payment plus any cost sharing) are equal to at least the total payment that would have been paid under Medicare fee-for-service, including any balance billing amounts.

D-10. What standards must Medicare Advantage plans meet for protection of beneficiaries?

In general, Medicare Advantage plans must meet standards similar to those related to disclosure, access, quality, grievances and appeals, confidentiality, and information on advance directives.

D-11. What are the rules regarding antidiscrimination?

Medicare Advantage plans cannot screen enrollees based on their health, nor can they discriminate with respect to participation, payment, or indemnification against any provider acting within the scope of the provider's license or certification. A Medicare Advantage plan, however, is not limited in its ability to selectively contract.

D-12. What are the rules regarding disclosure to enrollees?

A Medicare Advantage plan must provide in a clear, accurate, and standardized form certain information to each enrollee, such as the plan's service area, benefits, number, mix and distribution of providers, out-of-area coverage, emergency coverage, supplemental benefits, prior authorization rules, appeals and grievance procedures, and quality assurance program. Upon request, enrollees must be provided comparative information, information on the plan's utilization control mechanisms, information on the number of grievances and appeals, and compensation arrangements.

D-13. What are the access to services requirements for Medicare Advantage plans?

Medicare Advantage plans are permitted to select the providers who may furnish benefits to enrollees, as long as benefits are available and accessible to all enrollees with reasonable promptness and assured continuity, 24 hours a day, 7 days a week. The plan must also cover services provided other than through the organization for (1) non-emergency services needed immediately because of an unforeseen illness or injury, if it was not reasonable to obtain the services through the plan, (2) renal dialysis services for enrollees who are temporarily out of the plan's service area, and (3) maintenance or post-stabilization care after an emergency condition has been stabilized, subject to guidelines by the Centers for Medicare & Medicaid Services.

Medicare Advantage plans are required to pay for emergency services without regard to prior authorization or whether the provider has a contractual relationship with the plan. An emergency medical condition is defined using a "prudent layperson" standard (including conditions that may be manifested by "severe pain").

Private fee-for-service plans must demonstrate that the plan includes a sufficient number and range of providers willing to furnish services. This requirement is presumed to have been met if the plan has established payment rates that are not less than payment rates under Medicare, and/or has contracts or agreements with a sufficient number and range of providers.

D-14. Is there a quality assurance program for Medicare Advantage plans?

Medicare Advantage plans must have an internal quality assurance program. There are numerous requirements for internal quality assurance programs, but private fee-for-service plans must meet only a subset of those requirements, plus two requirements specific to those plans. Plans can meet internal quality assurance requirements by receiving accreditation from a private organization approved by Centers for Medicare & Medicaid Services. Medicare Advantage plans (except private fee-for-service plans that do not employ utilization review) must also undergo external quality reviews by QIOs or independent review organizations. Except in the case of the review of quality complaints, the Centers for Medicare & Medicaid Services is required to ensure that the external review activities are not duplicative of the review activities conducted as part of the accreditation process. The Centers for Medicare & Medicaid Services can waive external review requirements for organizations with good track records.

D-15. How are grievances handled by Medicare Advantage plans?

Medicare Advantage plans must maintain meaningful procedures for hearing and resolving grievances. Medicare Advantage plans must have a procedure for making determinations regarding whether an enrollee is entitled to receive services and the amount the individual is required to pay for such services. Determinations must be made on a timely basis. The explanation of a plan's determination must be in writing and must explain the reasons for the denial in understandable language and describe the reconsideration and appeals processes. The time period for reconsiderations will be specified by the Centers for Medicare & Medicaid Services (CMS) but must not be greater than 60 days after the request by the enrollee. Reconsiderations of coverage determinations to deny coverage based on lack of medical necessity must be made by a physician with expertise in the field of medicine which relates to the condition necessitating treatment.

Plans are required to have an expedited review process in cases where the normal time frame for making a determination or reconsideration could seriously jeopardize the life or health of the enrollee or the enrollee's ability to regain maximum function. Either the beneficiary or the physician can request an expedited review. Requests for expedited reviews made by physicians (even those not affiliated with the organization) must be granted by the plan. Expedited determinations and reconsiderations must be made within time periods specified by the CMS, but not later than 72 hours after the request for expedited review, or such longer period as the CMS may permit in specified cases.

The CMS is required to contract with an independent, outside entity to review and resolve plan reconsiderations not favorable to the beneficiary. If the independent review is unfavorable to the beneficiary, the beneficiary has the right to the same appeals process (e.g., Administrative Law Judge, judicial review) as under existing HMO procedures.

D-16. Are there special rules covering provider participation?

Yes, a Medicare Advantage plan must establish procedures relating to participation of physicians in the plan, such as notice of rules of participation, written notice of adverse participation decisions, and an appeals process. Medicare Advantage plans must consult with participating physicians regarding medical policy, quality, and medical management procedures.

Plans are prohibited from restricting health care professionals from advising their patients about the patient's health status or treatment options.

A provider, health professional, or other entity is treated as having a contract with a private fee-for-service plan if the provider, health professional, or other entity furnishes services that are covered under a private fee-for-service plan, and before providing those services, was informed of the individual's enrollment, and either was informed of the terms and conditions of payment for the services under the private fee-for-service plan or was given a reasonable opportunity to obtain information concerning the terms and conditions.

D-17. Are there billing limits under Medicare Advantage?

Non-contracting physicians and other entities must accept as payment in full the amount that would have been paid under Medicare fee-for-service. Non-contracting providers must also accept as payment in full, the amount that would have been paid under Medicare.

Contracting physicians, providers, and other entities of private fee-for-service plans must accept as payment in full an amount not to exceed (including any deductibles, coinsurance, copayments or balance billing permitted under the plan) an amount equal to 115% of the plan's payment rate. Plans must establish procedures to carry out this requirement. If a plan does not establish and enforce its procedures, the plan is subject to intermediate sanctions.

Private fee-for-service plans must provide enrollees with an explanation of benefits that includes a clear statement regarding enrollee liability, including any balance billing. The plan must also provide that the hospital give enrollees prior notice before they receive inpatient services and certain other services, when the amount of balance billing could be substantial. The notice must include a good faith estimate of the likely amount of balance billing based upon the presenting conditions of the enrollee.

PREMIUMS

D-18. How do Medicare Advantage plans submit proposed premiums?

All Medicare Advantage plans must submit to the Centers for Medicare & Medicaid Services (CMS) information on enrollment capacity. *Managed care plans* must submit adjusted community rate (ACR) proposals for basic and supplemental benefits, the plan's premium for the basic and supplemental benefits, a description of cost sharing, the actuarial value of cost sharing for basic and supplemental benefits, and a description of any additional benefits and the value of these benefits. *Private fee-for-service plans* must submit ACRs for basic and additional benefits, the premium for the basic and additional benefits, a description of cost sharing and the actuarial value of the cost sharing, a description of additional benefits and the actuarial value of these benefits, and the supplemental premium.

In general, CMS must review ACRs, premiums, and the actuarial values and approve or disapprove these rates, amounts, and values. But CMS will not review premiums of private fee-for-service plans.

Important: Organizations cannot contract to enroll Medicare beneficiaries under the Medicare Advantage program until they have met standards published by CMS.

D-19. What other premium rules should a beneficiary know about?

- A Medicare Advantage plan can terminate an enrollee for failure to pay premiums but only under specified conditions.

- A Medicare Advantage organization cannot offer cash or other monetary rebates as an inducement for enrollment or otherwise.

- Premiums cannot vary among plan enrollees.

- No state can impose a premium tax or similar tax on premiums of Medicare Advantage plans or the offering of these plans.

CONTRACTS WITH MEDICARE ADVANTAGE ORGANIZATIONS

D-20. How does a plan become part of the Medicare Advantage program?

A Medicare Advantage plan must generally be organized and licensed under state law as a risk bearing entity to offer health insurance or health benefits coverage.

Special rules formerly applied to Provider-Sponsored Organizations (PSOs). A PSO could seek a waiver from the requirement that it be licensed under state law by filing an application with the Centers for Medicare & Medicaid Services (CMS) no later than November 1, 2002. Waivers were effective for three years, were not applicable in any other state, and were not renewable.

New regional Preferred Provider Organizations are also eligible for temporary waiver of state licensure requirements. This is intended to facilitate the introduction of these multi-state plans. The CMS has indicated that it will grant these waivers only in cases where the organization is licensed in one state and has submitted applications in the other states. The length of the waiver will typically be for less than one year, but will depend on how long states take to process applications.

A plan cannot receive payment from Medicare unless it has a contract with the CMS. The contract period is for one year and may be automatically renewed in the absence of notice by either party of intention to terminate.

The CMS can terminate a contract if (1) the organization has failed to substantially carry out the contract, (2) the organization was carrying out the contract in a manner substantially inconsistent with the efficient and effective administration of the Medicare Advantage program, or (3) the organization no longer substantially meets Medicare Advantage conditions. The CMS may not contract with a plan that has been terminated within the last five years, except in special circumstances determined by the Administrator of the CMS.

Medicare Advantage plans must meet minimum enrollment requirements: 5,000 for plans in urban areas (1,500 for PSOs), 1,500 for plans in rural areas (500 for PSOs). These requirements can be waived in the first three contract years.

Medicare Advantage plans must provide prompt payment to non-contracting providers and to enrollees in the case of private fee-for-service plans. If the CMS determines (after notice of an opportunity for a hearing) that the plan has failed to pay providers or enrollees promptly, it can provide for direct payment. In these cases, the Centers for Medicare & Medicaid Services will reduce Medicare Advantage payments accordingly.

The CMS may impose intermediate sanctions if the plan (1) fails to provide medically necessary services required under law or the contract and the failure adversely affects or has the substantial likelihood of adversely affecting the enrollee, (2) imposes premiums in excess of the premium permitted, (3) acts to expel or refuses to re-enroll an individual in violation of the Medicare Advantage requirements, (4) engages in practices that effectively deny or discourage enrollment, (5) misrepresents or falsifies information to the CMS or to others, (6) violates rules regarding physician participation, (7) employs or contracts with individuals who are excluded from participation in Medicare, or (8) performs any other actions that are grounds for termination and, in the case of private fee-for-service plans, does not enforce balance billing limits. The remedies may include civil money penalties, suspension of enrollment, or suspension of payment.

Medicare Advantage plans must assume full financial risk for the provision of Medicare services except that plans can (1) obtain insurance or make other arrangements for costs in excess of amounts periodically determined by the Centers for Medicare & Medicaid Services; plans can obtain insurance or make arrangements for services needing to be provided other than through the plan, (2) obtain insurance or make other arrangements for not more than 90% of the amount by which its fiscal year costs exceeded 115% of its income for the year, (3) make arrangements with providers or health institutions to assume all or part of the risk on a prospective basis for the provision of basic services.

MEDIGAP INSURANCE PROGRAM

D-21. What rules apply regarding Medigap insurance and Medicare Advantage plans?

A Medigap insurance policy cannot be sold or issued to an individual with the knowledge that the policy duplicates health benefits to which the individual is entitled under the Medicare Advantage plan or another Medigap policy, unless accompanied by a written disclosure statement.

A Medicare Advantage plan is not considered a Medigap insurance policy. Medigap insurance policies supplement original fee-for-service Medicare coverage while a Medicare Advantage plan is an alternative to original fee-for-service Medicare coverage. See Section F for more information on Medigap insurance.

D-22. What are the special rules regarding Medigap protections under the Medicare Advantage program?

If an individual described below seeks to enroll in a Medigap policy within 63 days of the events described below, the issuer may not (1) deny or condition the issuance of a

Medigap policy that is offered or available, (2) discriminate in the pricing of a policy because of health status, claims experience, receipt of health care, or medical condition, and (3) impose a preexisting condition exclusion. See Section F for more information about Medigap insurance.

There is guaranteed issuance of Medigap insurance policies "A", "B", "C", or "F" for

(1) Individuals enrolled under an employee welfare benefit plan that provides benefits supplementing Medicare if the plan terminates or ceases to provide all benefits.

(2) Persons enrolled with a Medicare Advantage organization who discontinue under circumstances permitting disenrollment other than during an annual election period. These include (1) the termination of the entity's certification, (2) the individual moves outside the entity's service area, or (3) the individual elects termination due to cause.

(3) Persons enrolled with a risk or cost contract HMO, a similar organization operating under a demonstration project authority, a health care prepayment plan, or a Medicare SELECT policy, if enrollment ceases under the same circumstances that permit discontinuance of a Medicare Advantage election. In the case of a SELECT policy, there must also be no applicable provision in state law for continuation of the coverage.

(4) Individuals enrolled under a Medigap policy if enrollment ceases because of the bankruptcy or insolvency of the issuer, or because of other involuntary termination of coverage (and there is no provision under applicable state law for the continuation of coverage), or the issuer violated or misrepresented a provision of the policy.

There is guaranteed issuance of Medigap insurance plans "A", "B", "C", "F" or the Medigap insurance policy that the individual most recently previously enrolled in, if the individual (1) was enrolled under a Medigap policy, (2) subsequently terminates enrollment and enrolls with a Medicare Advantage organization, a risk or cost contract HMO, a similar organization operating under a demonstration project authority or a Medicare SELECT policy, and (3) terminates the Medicare Advantage enrollment within 12 months, but only if the individual was never previously enrolled with a Medicare Advantage organization.

There is guaranteed issuance of *any* Medigap plan to an individual who upon first becoming eligible for Medicare at age 65, enrolled in a Medicare Advantage plan, and disenrolled from the plan within 12 months of the effective date of enrollment.

PART D:

PRESCRIPTION DRUG INSURANCE

E-1. What is Medicare Part D?

Medicare Part D is the Prescription Drug Insurance program added to Medicare by the Medicare Prescription Drug, Improvement, and Modernization Act of 2003 (MMA).

Prescription Drug Insurance is a voluntary program of health insurance that covers a portion of prescription drug costs not generally covered by other Medicare programs. Prescription Drug Insurance is offered through private health plans. Participants may stay with traditional Medicare and enroll in a drug-only plan or may choose a Medicare Advantage plan with comprehensive benefits. Prescription Drug Insurance is partially financed through premiums paid by participants, whether for drug-only plans or as part of a Medicare Advantage premiums.

During the transition period before the Prescription Drug Insurance program was implemented, a Medicare drug discount card was available for a small annual enrollment fee.

E-2. When did Medicare Part D become effective?

The Part D Prescription Drug Insurance program was effective January 1, 2006. Initial open enrollment for Prescription Drug Insurance began November 15, 2005 and ran for six months to May 15, 2006. In 2006 and future years, open enrollment runs from November 15 to December 31 for the following benefit year. The enrollment periods for drug-only plans and Medicare Advantage plans run concurrently.

Beginning in May 2004 and continuing through December 31, 2005, Medicare recipients could enroll in the Medicare drug discount card program. Enrollment in the drug discount card program ended with the implementation of the Prescription Drug Insurance program.

E-3. Who is eligible for Medicare Part D?

Anyone who is entitled to Medicare Part A or enrolled in Part B is eligible to participate in Part D Prescription Drug Insurance. All Medicare participants were similarly eligible for the prescription drug discount card, excepting only those enrolled in Medicaid and entitled to Medicaid drug coverage.

E-4. What benefits did the Medicare drug discount card provide?

Medicare contracted with private companies to offer the voluntary drug discount cards. Medicare drug discount cards typically offered discounts ranging from 10% to 25% on prescription drugs. Not all pharmacies accepted all discount cards, and not all discount cards provided discounts on all drugs.

Individuals with income under 135% of the federal poverty level could qualify for a $600 credit on the discount card to pay for prescriptions. Individuals who already have drug coverage through Medicaid, TRICARE, or an employer group health plan are not eligible for the credit.

E-5. What did the Medicare drug discount card cost?

Medicare drug discount cards required an annual enrollment fee that could not exceed $30. Some cards were available at no cost.

The enrollment fee was waived for participants with income under 135% of the federal poverty level. These individuals also qualified for the $600 prescription drug credit.

E-6. What benefits does the Prescription Drug Insurance provide?

Prescription Drug Insurance offers a standard benefit to most participants. Participants with incomes below 135% and between 135% and 150% of the federal poverty guidelines will have lower cost sharing requirements than under the standard benefit.

Prescription Drug Insurance offers the following standard benefit in 2007:

Prescription Drug Expenses	Beneficiary Costs	Medicare Pays
First $265	100% (up to $265)	Nothing
$265-$2,400	25% (up to $533.75)	75% (up to $1,601.25)
$2,400-$5,451.25	100% (up to $3,051.25)	Nothing
Above $5,451.25	Up to 5% (based on income)	95% or more

Beneficiaries with incomes below 135% of the federal poverty guidelines have no cost-sharing obligation for prescription drug expenses above $5,100. Beneficiaries with incomes between 135% and 150% of the federal poverty guidelines have $2.15 and $5.35 co-pays for generic and name-brand prescriptions. Those with incomes above 150% of the federal poverty level have 5% co-pays.

For 2007, 135% of the federal poverty guidelines is $13,784 for a single person and $18,482 for a married couple; 150% of the federal poverty guidelines is $15,315 for a single person and $20,535 for a married couple. For 2006, 135% of the federal poverty guidelines was $13,230 for a single person and $17,820 for a married couple; 150% of the federal poverty guidelines was $14,700 for a single person and $19,800 for a married couple.

Sponsoring organizations may offer alternative prescription drug coverage through plans that (1) provide coverage, the actuarial value of which is at least equal to the actuarial value of the standard prescription drug coverage, (2) offer access to negotiated prices, and (3) are approved by CMS.

Part D plans may also provide supplemental prescription drug coverage that offers cost-sharing reductions and optional drugs. A plan may charge a supplemental premium for the supplemental coverage. But a sponsoring organization offering supplemental coverage in an area must also offer a prescription drug plan in the area that provides only basic coverage for no additional supplemental premium. Basic coverage is either the statutorily-defined standard benefit or the alternative prescription drug coverage without any supplemental benefits.

E-7. What does the Prescription Drug Insurance cost?

Medicare Prescription Drug Insurance requires payment of a monthly premium averaging approximately $27.35 in 2007. The premium may be paid separately for a drug-only plan or as part of the premium for a comprehensive Medicare Advantage Plan.

Beneficiaries who choose not to enroll in Prescription Drug Insurance during their initial enrollment period may face a late enrollment penalty if they later choose to enter the program. The late enrollment penalty is the greater of "an amount that [CMS] determines is actuarially sound for each uncovered month" or "1 percent of the base beneficiary premium" (the national average premium for the year of late enrollment) per month. (This penalty is similar to the penalty currently in place for late enrollment in Medicare Part B, 10 percent per 12-month period.) For those enrolling in 2007, the penalty will be approximately $0.27 per full month in which they were eligible to enroll in Prescription Drug Insurance but did not.

Beneficiaries who have other sources of drug coverage may be able to maintain that coverage and not enroll in Prescription Drug Insurance without penalty. If a beneficiary's existing coverage is at least as good as Prescription Drug Insurance (i.e., considered "creditable coverage") then the beneficiary can avoid any late enrollment penalties if he later enrolls in Prescription Drug Insurance. Creditable coverage must be actuarially equivalent to Part D Prescription Drug Insurance. Failure to maintain creditable prescription drug coverage for a period of 63 days or long may subject an individual to a later enrollment penalty.

Entities (such as a former employer) offering prescription drug coverage to Part D eligible individuals must disclose to those individuals whether the coverage they provide is creditable coverage as defined by CMS. These entities must also inform CMS of the status of this coverage. See E-8.

E-8. What notice must an employer who maintains an accident or health plan provide to Medicare-eligible individuals?

Employers and plan sponsors who offer prescription drug coverage to individuals eligible for Medicare Part D must advise those individuals whether the offered coverage is "creditable." Eligible individuals who do not enroll in Part D when first available, but who enroll later, have to pay higher premiums permanently, unless they have creditable prescription drug coverage. See E-7.

To determine that coverage is creditable, a sponsor need only determine that total expected paid claims for Medicare beneficiaries under the sponsor's plan will be at least equal to the total expected paid claims for the same beneficiaries under the defined standard prescription drug coverage under Part D. The determination of creditable coverage status for disclosure purposes does not require attestation by a qualified actuary (unless the employer or union is applying for the retiree drug subsidy available under the MMA).

To assist sponsors in making the determination that coverage is creditable, the Center for Medicare & Medicaid Studies (CMS) issued guidance with example "safe harbor" benefit designs. A plan design will automatically be deemed creditable if it includes

1. coverage for brand and generic prescriptions;

2. reasonable access to retail providers and, optionally, for mail order coverage;

3. benefits payments designed to pay on average at least 60% of participants' prescription drug expenses; and

4. at least one of the following:

    a. an annual prescription drug benefit maximum of at least $25,000,

    b. an actuarial expectation that the plan will pay benefits of at least $2,000 per Medicare-eligible individual, or

    c. for plans that cover both medical expenses and prescription drugs, an annual deductible of no more than $250, an annual benefit maximum of at least $25,000, and a lifetime maximum of at least $1,000,000.

Under the CMS guidance, once a sponsor determines whether coverage is creditable, the sponsor must provide notice to all Part D-eligible individuals covered by or applying for the plan, including Part D-eligible dependents. In lieu of determining who is Part D eligible, an employer sponsor may provide notice to all active employees, along with an explanation of why the notice is being provided.

The required notice to beneficiaries must, at a minimum,

1. contain a statement that the employer has determined that the coverage is creditable (or not creditable),

2. explain the meaning of creditable coverage,

3. explain why creditable coverage is important, and caution that higher Part D premiums could result if there is a break in creditable coverage of 63 days or more before enrolling in a Part D plan, and

4. if coverage is not creditable, explain that an individual may generally enroll in Part D only from November 15 through December 31 of each year.

CMS recommends that sponsors also provide the following clarifications in their notice:

- An explanation of a beneficiary's rights to a notice, i.e., the times when a beneficiary can expect to receive a notice and the times that a beneficiary can request a copy of the notice.

- An explanation of the plan provisions that affect beneficiaries when they (or their dependent) are Medicare Part D eligible. These options may include, for example

  o that they can retain their existing coverage and choose not to enroll in a Part D plan; or

  o that they can enroll in a Part D plan as a supplement to, or in lieu of, the other coverage.

  o If their existing prescription drug coverage is under a Medigap policy, that they cannot have both their existing prescription drug coverage and Part D coverage, and that if they enroll in Part D coverage, they should inform their Medigap insurer of that fact, and the Medigap insurer must remove the prescription drug coverage from the Medigap policy and adjust the premium, as of the date the Part D coverage starts.

- Whether the covered individuals and/or their covered dependents will still be eligible to receive all of their current health coverage if they or their dependent enrolls in a Medicare prescription drug plan.

- A clarification of the circumstances (if any) under which the individual could re-enroll in his prescription drug coverage if he drops the current coverage and enrolls in Medicare prescription drug coverage. (For Medigap insurers, this would be a clarification that the individual cannot get his prescription drug coverage back under such circumstances).

- Information on how to get extra help paying for a Medicare prescription drug plan including the contact information for the Social Security Administration (SSA).

The CMS guidance includes model initial notices and suggested language that a sponsor may choose to use. Sponsors were required to provide initial notices to all beneficiaries by November 15, 2005. The guidance and model notices are available on the CMS website at http://www.cms.hhs.gov/creditablecoverage.

Sponsors must also disclose to CMS whether the coverage is creditable. The disclosure must be made to CMS on an annual basis, and upon any change that affects whether the coverage is creditable. CMS has posted guidance on the timing and format of the required disclosure and a model Disclosure to CMS form on the CMS website at http://www.cms. hhs.gov/creditablecoverage.

MEDIGAP INSURANCE

F-1. What is Medigap Insurance?

Medicare provides basic protection against the cost of health care, but it does not pay all medical expenses or most long-term care expenses. For this reason, many private insurance companies sell supplement (Medigap) insurance as well as separate long-term care insurance. The federal government does not sell or service insurance, but regulates the coverage offered by Medigap insurance.

Medigap insurance is a private insurance policy designed to help pay deductibles or coinsurance incurred by beneficiaries who are in the original Medicare plan (also called fee-for-service Medicare). A Medigap policy may also pay for certain items or services not covered by Medicare at all, such as prescription drugs. Medigap only works with the original Medicare plan. It will not cover out-of-pocket expenses, such as copayments, in a managed care plan.

The majority of Medicare's elderly beneficiaries using fee-for-service have private Medigap policies. However, most of the elderly enrolled in managed care plans do not have any other type of coverage.

F-2. Is there an open enrollment period for Medigap policies?

Yes, an open enrollment period for selecting Medigap policies guarantees that for six months immediately following the effective date of enrolling in Medicare Part B, a person age 65 or older cannot be denied Medigap insurance or charged higher premiums because of health problems.

No matter how a person enrolls in Medicare Medical Insurance—whether by automatic notification or through an initial, special or general enrollment period—a person is covered by the guarantees if both of the following are true:

- The person is age 65 or older and is enrolled in Medicare for the first time, based on age rather than disability.

- The person applies for Medigap insurance within six months of enrollment in Medical Insurance (Part B).

But note that even when a person buys a Medigap policy in this open enrollment period, the policy may still exclude coverage for "pre-existing conditions" during the first six months the policy is in effect. Pre-existing conditions are conditions that were either diagnosed or treated during the six-month period before the Medigap policy became effective. (See F-3 for exceptions to this rule.)

Once the Medigap open enrollment period ends, a person may not be able to buy the policy of his choice. He may have to accept whatever Medigap policy an insurance company is willing to sell him.

In the case of individuals enrolled in Medicare Part B prior to age 65, Medigap insurers are required to offer coverage, regardless of medical history, for a six-month period when the individual reaches age 65. Insurers are prohibited from discriminating in the price of policies for such an individual, based upon the medical or health status of the policyholder.

Also, although Medigap policies are standardized, premiums can vary widely. Insurers can reject an applicant who applies for a Medigap policy after the open enrollment period.

All Medigap polices are guaranteed renewable. This means that they continue in force as long as the premium is paid.

F-3. Does a Medicaid recipient need Medigap insurance?

Low-income people who are eligible for Medicaid usually do not need additional insurance. Medicaid pays for certain health care benefits beyond those covered by Medicare, such as long-term nursing home care. If a person purchases Medigap insurance and later becomes eligible for Medicaid, he can ask that the Medigap insurance benefits and premiums be suspended for up to two years while he is covered by Medicaid. If the person becomes ineligible for Medicaid benefits during the two years, the Medigap policy is automatically reinstated provided the person gives proper notice and begins paying premiums again.

F-4. Are there federal standards for Medigap policies?

Yes, Congress established federal standards for Medigap policies in 1990. Most states have adopted regulations limiting the sale of Medigap insurance to no more than 12 standard policies. One of the 12 is a basic policy offering a "core package" of benefits. These standardized plans are identified by the letters A through L. Plan A is the core package. Plans B through J each have a different combination of benefits, but they all include the core package. Plans K and L, new in 2006, do not include the core benefit package. They instead offer catastrophic coverage. The basic policy, offering the core package of benefits, is available in all states. The availability of other plans varies from state to state.

The core package of benefits which all policies A through J must contain includes the following benefits:

- Hospital Insurance (Part A) coinsurance for the 61st through 90th day of hospitalization in any Medicare benefit period,

- Hospital Insurance coinsurance for the 91st through 150th day,

- Hospital Insurance expenses for an extra 365 days in the hospital,

- Hospital Insurance (Part A) and Medical Insurance (Part B) deductible for the cost of the first three pints of blood, and

- Medical Insurance (Part B) coinsurance (20% of allowable charges).

F-5. What additional benefits can be offered in the standard Medigap plans?

The following additional benefits above the basic core benefits can be covered:

- The entire $992 Hospital Insurance deductible.

- The $124.00 a day coinsurance for days 21-100 of skilled nursing home care under Hospital Insurance.

- The $131 Medical Insurance deductible.

- 80% of the "balance billing" paid by Medical Insurance beneficiaries whose doctors do not accept assignment.

- 100% of lawful balance billing.

- 80% of the Medicare-eligible costs of medically necessary emergency care when the insured is traveling outside the United States.

- Up to $120 a year for certain screening and preventive measures.

- Certain "short term, at-home assistance with activities of daily living" for people recovering from illness, injury, or surgery at home, in a relative's home, or in an institution (but not a hospital or skilled nursing facility), up to $1,600 a year, with not more than seven four-hour visits by caregivers in any week, with no more than $40 reimbursement per visit. The care must be received while the person is getting Medicare home care (or within eight weeks of the termination of Medicare home care)—but visits paid for by Medicare or other government programs cannot be covered under a Medigap policy; nor can care be provided by family members or unpaid volunteers.

- "Innovative benefits" that are appropriate, cost-effective, and consistent with the goal of simplifying Medigap insurance—with prior approval by the state insurance commissioner.

- 50% of outpatient prescription drug costs, subject to a $250 deductible with an annual maximum of $1,250 ("basic prescription drug benefit"). (*This may no longer be offered to new customers.*)

- 50% of outpatient prescription drug costs, with a $250 deductible and a $3,000 annual maximum ("extended prescription drug benefit"). (*This may no longer be offered to new customers.*)

F-6. What benefits are provided in each of the standard Medigap policies and the high deductible Medigap policies?

The Medigap policies offer the following benefits:

- Policy A is the basic core benefit package. (See F-4.)

- Policy B includes: (1) the basic core benefit package, and (2) the Hospital Insurance (Part A) deductible ($992 in 2007).

- Policy C includes: (1) the basic core benefit package, (2) the Hospital Insurance (Part A) deductible ($992 in 2007), (3) the coinsurance for care in a skilled nursing home (days 21-100, $124 per day in 2007), (4) the Medical Insurance (Part B) deductible ($131 in 2007), and (5) coverage of foreign travel emergencies.

- Policy D includes: (1) the basic core benefit package, (2) the Hospital Insurance (Part A) deductible ($992 in 2007), (3) the coinsurance for care in a skilled nursing home (days 21-100, $124 a day in 2007), (4) coverage of foreign travel emergencies, and (5) at-home recovery assistance.

- Policy E includes: (1) the basic core benefit package, (2) the Hospital Insurance (Part A) deductible ($992 in 2007), (3) the coinsurance for care in a skilled nursing home (days 21-100, $124 a day in 2007), (4) coverage of foreign travel emergencies, and (5) coverage of preventive screening and care.

- Policy F includes: (1) the basic core benefit package, (2) the Hospital Insurance (Part A) deductible ($992 in 2007), (3) the coinsurance for care in a skilled nursing home (days 21-100, $124 a day in 2007), (4) the Medical Insurance (Part B) deductible ($131 in 2007), (5) coverage of foreign travel emergencies, and (6) 100% coverage of excess doctor charges under Medical Insurance (Part B).

- Policy G includes: (1) the basic core benefit package, (2) the Hospital Insurance (Part A) deductible ($992 in 2007), (3) the coinsurance for care in a skilled nursing home (days 21-100, $124 a day in 2007), (4) coverage of foreign travel emergencies, (5) at-home recovery assistance, and (6) 80% of excess doctor charges under Medical Insurance (Part B).

- Policy H includes: (1) the basic core benefit package, (2) the Hospital Insurance (Part A) deductible ($992 in 2007), (3) the coinsurance for care in a skilled nursing home (days 21-100, $124 a day in 2007), (4) coverage of foreign travel emergencies, and (5) coverage of 50% of the cost of outpatient prescription drugs after payment of a $250 deductible, up to a maximum benefit of $1,250. (But see the note below regarding prescription drug coverage.)

- Policy I includes: (1) the basic core benefit package, (2) the Hospital Insurance (Part A) deductible ($992 in 2007), (3) the coinsurance for care in a skilled nursing home (days 21-100, $124 a day in 2007), (4) coverage of foreign travel emergencies, (5) at-home recovery assistance, (6) 100% of excess doctor charges under Medical Insurance (Part B), and (7) 50% of the cost of outpatient prescription drugs after payment of a $250 deductible, up to a maximum benefit of $1,250. (But see the note below regarding prescription drug coverage.)

- Policy J includes: (1) the basic core benefit package, (2) the Hospital Insurance (Part A) deductible ($992 in 2007), (3) the coinsurance for care in a skilled nursing home (days 21-100, $124 a day in 2007), (4) the Medical Insurance (Part B) deductible ($131 in 2007), (5) coverage of foreign travel emergencies, (6) at-home recovery assistance, (7) 100% of excess doctor charges under Medical Insurance (Part B), (8) preventive screening and care, and (9) 50% of the cost of outpatient prescription drugs after payment of a $250 deductible, up to a maximum benefit of $3,000. (But see the note below regarding prescription drug coverage.)

- There is a policy that is the same as Policy F but with a $1, 860 deductible (in 2007). This high deductible policy covers 100% of covered out-of-pocket expenses once the deductible has been satisfied in a year. It requires the beneficiary of the policy to pay annual out-of-pocket expenses (other than premiums) in the amount of $1,860 before the policy begins payment of benefits. The deductible increases by the percentage increase in the Consumer Price Index for all urban consumers for the 12-month period ending with August of the preceding year.

- There is also a policy that is the same as Policy J but with a $1, 860 deductible (in 2007). This high deductible policy covers 100% of covered out-of-pocket expenses once the deductible has been satisfied in a year. It requires the beneficiary of the policy to pay annual out-of-pocket expenses (other than premiums) in the amount of $1,860 before the policy begins payment of benefits.

Note: As of January 1, 2006, beneficiaries who hold standard policies H, I, or J may choose between enrolling in Part D or maintaining their prescription drug coverage under their Medigap policies. Beneficiaries who choose to enroll in Part D may keep their existing plan H, I, or J, less the prescription drug benefit, or may purchase a new Medigap policy. As of January 1, 2006, plans H, I, and J may still be sold, but without the prescription drug benefit.

Beginning in 2006, two new standard plans were available. These two plans do not include the entire core benefit package.

- New Plan K includes (1) coverage of 50% of the cost-sharing otherwise applicable under Parts A and B, except for the Part B deductible, (2) coverage of 100% of hospital inpatient coinsurance and 365 extra lifetime days of coverage of inpatient hospital services, (3) coverage of 100% of any cost-sharing otherwise applicable for preventive benefits, and (4) a limit on annual out-of-pocket spending under Part A and Part B to $4,140 (in 2007).

- New Plan L includes (1) coverage of 75% of the cost-sharing otherwise applicable under Parts A and B, except for the Part B deductible, (2) coverage of 100% of hospital inpatient coinsurance and 365 extra lifetime days of coverage of inpatient hospital services, (3) coverage of 100% of any cost-sharing otherwise applicable for preventive benefits, and (4) a limit on annual out-of-pocket spending under Part A and Part B to $2,070 (in 2007).

Some choices may not be available in Massachusetts, Minnesota, and Wisconsin because these states already required standardized Medigap policies prior to 1992.

F-7. What are Medicare SELECT policies?

The difference between Medicare SELECT and regular Medigap insurance is that a Medicare SELECT policy may (except in emergencies) limit Medigap benefits to items and services provided by certain selected health care professionals or may pay only partial benefits when the patient gets health care from other health care professionals.

Insurers, including some HMOs, offer Medicare SELECT in the same way they offer standard Medigap insurance. The policies are required to meet certain federal standards and are regulated by the states in which they are approved. A person is able to choose from among the 10 Medigap policies, but the premiums charged for Medicare SELECT policies are generally lower than premiums for comparable Medigap policies that do not have this selected-provider feature.

State insurance departments have information about Medicare SELECT policies that have been approved for sale in their states.

F-8. Should a person purchase the most comprehensive policy if he can afford the premiums?

Not necessarily. A person must determine which benefits he is likely to need before purchasing a Medigap policy. Often, a person does not need the most comprehensive policy.

For example, Policy A is the least expensive policy and offers the basic core package of benefits. Policies F and G might be considered if a person uses nonparticipating doctors—those who charge more than the amount approved by Medicare; however, excess charges are limited to 115% of what Medicare pays (see C-11). If the doctors charge no more than the amount approved by Medicare, less expensive policies such as Policy C or Policy D may be appropriate. Policy D also includes important benefits not covered by Policy A, such as coverage of custodial care at home following an illness or injury and the cost of coinsurance for skilled nursing home care.

F-9. What Medigap insurance protections are there for those enrolled in the Medicare Advantage program?

For many years Medicare law allowed for Medicare covered services to be furnished to individuals through HMOs that contracted with Medicare. The Medicare Advantage program was created by Congress in 1997. Medicare Advantage expands the types of health plans that can contract with Medicare to enroll beneficiaries.

A person who currently has a Medigap policy may enroll in a Medicare Advantage plan and can keep the Medigap policy after enrollment. Keeping the Medigap policy may give a person time to determine whether to stay in the Medicare Advantage plan or return to the original Medicare plan with Medigap insurance. However, expenses paid for by the Medicare Advantage plan will not be reimbursed by the Medigap insurer. Eventually the person should drop Medigap coverage if satisfied with the Medicare Advantage plan.

A person already enrolled in a Medicare Advantage plan cannot buy Medigap insurance but may have the right to purchase a Medigap policy by returning to the original fee-for-service Medicare plan. To be guaranteed the right to buy Medigap insurance the person must have enrolled in the Medicare Advantage plan at age 65, must terminate enrollment in the Medicare Advantage plan within 12 months of entry into that plan, and must not have had any previous enrollment in a Medicare managed care plan.

If a Medicare Advantage plan terminates coverage because it leaves the Medicare program, plan enrollees have certain rights to new coverage, but these are time limited. The Medicare Advantage plan is required to provide information to assist making a decision about enrolling in another Medicare Advantage plan or switching to the original Medicare plan with a Medigap policy to supplement the coverage. In general, most individuals with Medicare have the right to guaranteed issue of any Medigap policies designated A, B, C, or F that are offered to new enrollees by issuers in the state.

This right applies to individuals by virtue of the involuntary termination of their coverage. However, certain Medicare beneficiaries in terminating Medicare Advantage plans may have another basis for entitlement to guaranteed issue of a Medigap policy. If a person had been enrolled in the Medicare Advantage plan for fewer than 12 months, was never enrolled in any other Medicare HMO, and had a previous Medigap policy, that person may return to the former Medigap policy if the previous Medigap insurance company still sells the policy in the state.

If that coverage is not available under the previous Medigap policy, the individual may purchase Medigap polices A, B, C, or F from any insurer who sells these policies in the state.

The insurance company selling the policy may not (1) deny or condition the sale of the policy, (2) discriminate in the pricing of the policy because of health status, prior history of claims experience, receipt of health care for a medical condition, or (3) impose an exclusion for any pre-existing condition.

But the individual has only 63 days after coverage ends to select a Medigap insurer. Also, if the individual moves outside the Medicare Advantage plan's service area, he has 63 days to select a Medigap insurer.

An individual is guaranteed issuance of *any* Medigap policy if (1) at least 65 years old, (2) eligible for Medicare, (3) enrolled in a Medicare Advantage plan, and (4) disenrolled from that plan within 12 months of the effective date of enrollment.

See SECTION D for a complete description of Medicare Advantage (Part C).

F-10. Are there rules for selling Medigap insurance?

Yes, both state and federal laws govern sales of Medigap insurance. Companies or agents selling Medigap insurance must avoid certain illegal practices.

It is unlawful to sell or issue to an individual entitled to benefits under Hospital Insurance (Part A) or enrolled under Medical Insurance (Part B) (1) a health insurance policy with knowledge that the policy duplicates health benefits the individual is otherwise entitled to under Medicare or Medicaid, (2) a Medigap policy with knowledge that the individual is entitled to benefits under another Medigap policy, or (3) a health insurance policy, other than a Medigap policy, with knowledge that the policy duplicates health benefits to which the individual is otherwise entitled.

Penalties do not apply, however, to the sale or issuance of a policy or plan that duplicates health benefits to which the individual is otherwise entitled if, under the policy or plan, all benefits are fully payable directly to or on behalf of the individual without regard to other health benefit coverage of the individual. In addition, for the penalty to be waived in the case of the sale or issuance of a policy or plan that duplicates benefits under Medicare or Medicaid, the application for the policy must include a statement, prominently displayed, disclosing the extent to which benefits payable under the policy or plan duplicate Medicare benefits.

The National Association of Insurance Commissioners (NAIC) has identified 10 separate types of health insurance policies that must provide an individualized statement of the extent to which the policy duplicates Medicare. These policies include the following:

- Policies that provide benefits for expenses incurred for an accidental injury only

- Policies that provide benefits for specified limited services

- Policies that reimburse expenses incurred for specified disease or other specific impairments (including cancer policies, specified disease policies and other policies that limit reimbursement to named medical conditions)

- Policies that pay fixed dollar amounts for specified disease or other specified impairments (including cancer, specified disease policies and other policies that pay a scheduled benefit or specified payment based on diagnosis of the conditions named in the policy)

- Indemnity policies and other policies that pay a fixed dollar amount per day, excluding long-term care policies

- Policies that provide benefits for both expenses incurred and fixed indemnity

- Long-term care policies providing both nursing home and non-institutional coverage

- Long-term care policies primarily providing nursing home benefits only

- Home care policies

- Other health insurance policies not specifically identified above

Certain policies are *not* required to carry a disclosure statement: (1) policies that do not duplicate Medicare benefits, even incidentally, (2) life insurance policies that contain long term care riders or accelerated death benefits, (3) disability insurance policies, (4) property and casualty policies, (5) employer and union group health plans, (6) managed care organizations with Medicare contracts, and (7) health care prepayment plans (HCPPs) that provide some or all Medicare Part B benefits under an agreement with the Centers for Medicare & Medicaid Services.

Policies offering only long-term care nursing home care, home health care, or community based care, or any combination of the three, are allowed to coordinate benefits with Medicare and are not considered duplicative, provided the coordination is disclosed.

An insurer is subject to civil money and criminal penalties for failing to provide the appropriate disclosure statement. Federal criminal and civil penalties (fines) may also be imposed against any insurance company or agent that knowingly

- sells a health insurance policy that duplicates a person's Medicare or Medicaid coverage, or any private health insurance coverage the person may have;

- tells a person that they are employees or agents of the Medicare program or of any government agency;

- makes a false statement that a policy meets legal standards for certification when it does not;

- sells a person a Medigap policy that is not one of the 10 approved standard policies (after the new standards have been put in place in the person's state);

- denies a person his Medigap open enrollment period by refusing to issue the person a policy, placing conditions on the policy, or discriminating in the price of a policy because of the person's health status, claims experience, receipt of health care, or the person's medical condition; or

- uses the United States mail in a state for advertising or delivering health insurance policies to supplement Medicare if the policies have not been approved for sale in that state.

The sale of a Medigap policy to a Medicaid beneficiary is prohibited. There is no prohibition on sale of policies to low-income Medicare beneficiaries for whom Medicaid pays only the Medical Insurance (Part B) premiums. As of January 1, 2006, plans H, I, and J may still be sold, but without the prescription drug benefit. See F-6.

F-11. What should a consumer be aware of when shopping for Medigap insurance?

The Centers for Medicare & Medicaid Services offers the following suggestions when shopping for Medigap insurance:

(1) *Review the plans.* The benefits in each of the standardized Medigap policies are the same no matter which insurance company sells it. Review the plans and choose the benefits that you need most.

(2) *Shop carefully before you buy.* Although each of the standardized Medigap policies is the same no matter which insurance company sells it, the costs may be very different. Companies use different ways to price Medigap policies. Companies

also differ in customer service. Call different insurance companies and compare cost and service before you buy.

(3)   *Don't buy more than one Medigap policy at a time.* It is illegal for an insurance company to sell you a second Medigap policy unless you tell them in writing that you are going to cancel the first Medigap policy when the second Medigap policy goes into effect. You should report anyone who tries to sell you a Medigap policy when you already have one.

(4)   *Check for pre-existing conditions exclusions.* Before you buy a Medigap policy, you should find out whether it has a waiting period before it fully covers your pre-existing conditions. If you have a health problem that was diagnosed or treated during the six months immediately before the Medigap policy starts, the policy might not cover your costs right away for care related to that health problem. Medigap policies must cover pre-existing conditions after the policy has been in effect for six months. Some insurance companies may have shorter waiting periods before covering a pre-existing condition. Other insurance companies may not have any waiting period. If you buy a policy during your Medigap open enrollment period, the insurance company must shorten the waiting period for pre-existing conditions by the amount of previous health coverage you have.

(5)   *Be careful of switching from one Medigap policy to another.* You should only switch policies to get different benefits, better service, or a better price. However, do not keep a policy that does not meet your needs because you have had it for a long time. If you decide to buy a new Medigap policy, the company must count the time you had the same benefits under the first policy towards the pre-existing conditions waiting period. However, you may have a waiting period for pre-existing conditions for new benefits that you did not have under your first policy. You must also sign a statement that you plan to cancel the first policy. Do not cancel the first policy until you are sure that you want to keep the new policy. You have 30 days to decide if you want to keep the new policy. This is called your free look period.

(6)   *Make sure you get your policy within 30 days.* You should get your policy within 30 days. If you do not, call the company and ask them to put in writing why the policy was delayed. If 60 days go by without an answer, call your State Insurance Department.

(7)   *Watch out for illegal marketing practices.* It is illegal for an insurance company or agent to pressure you into buying a Medigap policy, or lie to you or mislead you to get you to switch from one company or policy to another. False advertising is also illegal. Another type of illegal advertising involves mailing cards to people who may want to buy insurance. If you fill out and return the card enclosed in the mailing, the card may be sold to an insurance agent who will try to sell you a policy.

(8)   *Neither the state nor federal government sells or services Medigap policies.* State Insurance Departments approve Medigap policies sold by private insurance companies. This means that the company and Medigap policy meet requirements

of state law. Do not believe statements that Medigap insurance is a government-sponsored program. It is illegal for anyone to tell you that they are from the government and try to sell you a Medigap policy. If this happens to you, report that person to your State Insurance Department. It is also illegal for a company or agent to claim that a Medigap policy has been approved for sale in any state in which it has not been.

(9) *Find out if the insurance company is licensed.* An insurance company must meet certain standards in order to sell policies in your state. You should check with your State Insurance Department to make sure that the insurance company you are doing business with is licensed in your state. This is for your protection. Insurance agents must also be licensed by your state and the state may require them to carry proof that they are licensed. The proof will show their name and the name of the companies they represent. Do not buy a policy from any insurance agent that cannot prove that he or she is licensed. A business card is not a license.

(10) *Start looking early so you won't be rushed.* Do not be pressured into buying a Medigap policy. Good sales people will not rush you. Keep in mind, that if you are within your 6-month Medigap open enrollment period or in a situation where you have a guaranteed right to buy a Medigap policy, there are time limits you must follow. Buying the Medigap policy of your choice may be harder after the Medigap open enrollment or special protection period ends. This will be especially true if you have a pre-existing health condition. If you are not sure whether a Medigap policy is what you need, ask the salesperson to explain it to you with a friend or family member present.

(11) *Keep agents' and/or companies' names, addresses, and telephone numbers.* Write down the agents' and/or companies' names, addresses, and telephone numbers or ask for a business card with this information.

(12) *If you decide to buy, fill out the application carefully.* Do not believe an insurance agent who says your medical history on an application is not important. Some companies ask for detailed medical information. You must answer the medical questions even if you are applying during your Medigap open enrollment period or are in a situation where you have the right to buy a Medigap policy. During these two times, the company cannot use your answers to turn you down or use this information to decide how much to charge you for a Medigap policy. However, if you leave out any of the medical information they ask for, the company could refuse to cover you for a period of time for any medical condition you did not report. The company also could deny a claim or cancel your Medigap policy if you send in a bill for care of a health problem you did not report.

(13) *Beware of non-standardized plans.* It is illegal for anyone to sell you a policy and call it a Medigap policy if it does not match the standardized Medigap policies sold in your state. A doctor may offer you a "retainer agreement" that says he/she can provide certain non-Medicare-covered services and not charge you the Medicare coinsurance and deductible amounts. This type of agreement may be illegal. If a doctor refuses to see you as a Medicare patient unless you pay

him or her a yearly fee and sign a "retainer agreement," you should call 1-800-MEDICARE.

(14) *Look for an outline of coverage*. You must be given a clearly worded summary of a Medigap policy. Read it carefully.

(15) *Do not pay cash*. Pay by check, money order, or bank draft payable to the insurance company, not the agent or anyone else. Get a receipt with the insurance company's name, address, and telephone number for your records.

HOW TO SUBMIT CLAIMS AND APPEALS

CLAIMS PROCEDURE

G-1. How does Medicare pay for Hospital Insurance (Part A) services?

Hospital Insurance helps pay for covered services received in a hospital or skilled nursing facility or from a home health agency or hospice program. Hospitals, skilled nursing facilities, home health agencies and hospices are called "providers" under the Hospital Insurance program. Providers submit their claims directly to Medicare. The patient cannot submit claims for services. The provider will charge the patient for any part of the Hospital Insurance deductible he has not met and any coinsurance he owes. Providers cannot require the patient to make a deposit before being admitted for inpatient care that is or may be covered under Hospital Insurance.

Intermediaries process claims submitted on the patient's behalf by hospitals, skilled nursing facilities, home health agencies, hospices and certain other providers of services. When the Medicare intermediary pays a claim, the patient gets a *Notice of Medicare Benefit*. This notice is not a bill.

G-2. How does a person submit Medical Insurance (Part B) claims?

Doctors, suppliers, and other providers of Medical Insurance services are in most cases required to submit Medicare claims for the patient even if they do not take assignment. They must submit the claims by December 31 of the following year for services furnished during the first nine months of the year. Claims must be submitted by December 31 of the second following year for services furnished during the last three months of the year. A patient should notify the Medicare carrier if the doctor or supplier refuses to submit a Medical Insurance claim and the patient believes the services may be covered by Medicare.

The doctor or supplier must submit a form, called a CMS-1500 requesting that a Medical Insurance payment be made for the patient's covered services, whether or not assignment is taken. The doctor or supplier completes form CMS-1500. (Ambulance services previously submitted claims on CMS-1491, but on or after April 2, 2007, they are required to submit claims on CMS-1500.) The patient must sign the form before the doctor or supplier sends it to the proper Medicare carrier. If a patient's claim is for the rental or purchase of durable medical equipment, a doctor's prescription or certificate of medical necessity must be included with the claim.

If the patient is enrolled in a coordinated care plan such as an HMO, a claim will seldom need to be submitted on the patient's behalf. Medicare pays the HMO a set amount and the HMO provides the patient's medical care. Physicians, supplies and other providers of Medical Insurance services bill the HMO to receive payment for their services at a contractually-agreed rate.

After the doctor, provider, or supplier sends in a Medical Insurance claim, Medicare will send the patient a notice called *Explanation of Your Medicare Part B Benefits* to tell the patient the decision on the claim. The notice gives the address and toll-free number for contacting the carrier.

The carrier pays 80% of the amount determined to be the reasonable charge or set by a fee schedule. The patient must pay the 20% balance. In addition, the carrier will withhold from the patient the amount of the annual deductible ($131).

Payment can be made directly to the doctor or supplier. This is the *assignment method*. The doctor or supplier is prohibited from charging the patient anything above the 20% coinsurance amount and the amount of the patient's deductible if the deductible has not been paid. Medicare pays the doctor or supplier 80% of the reasonable charge.

G-3. What must an itemized bill contain?

The itemized bill must show (1) the date the patient received the services, (2) the place where the patient received the services, (3) a description of the services, (4) the charge for each service, (5) the doctor or supplier who provided the services, and (6) the patient's name and health insurance claim number, including the letter at the end of the number.

If the bill does not contain all of this information, payment may be delayed. It is also helpful if the nature of the patient's illness (diagnosis) is shown on the bill.

A doctor or supplier submitting a claim for the rental or purchase of durable medical equipment should include the bill from his prescription. The prescription must show the equipment needed, the medical reason for the need, and estimate how long the equipment will be medically necessary.

Before any Medical Insurance (Part B) payment can be made, a person's record must show that he has met the $131 (in 2007) deductible. Once a person has met the deductible, his doctor or supplier should send in future bills for covered services as soon as possible so that Medicare payment can be made promptly. If all medical bills for the year amount to less than the deductible, Medical Insurance cannot pay any part of a person's bills for the year.

G-4. What happens if the patient dies and payments are due?

Hospital Insurance payments due will be paid directly to the hospital, skilled nursing facility, home health agency or hospice that provided covered services.

Special rules apply for services covered under Medical Insurance. If the bill was paid by the patient or with funds from the patient's estate, payment will be made either to the estate representative or to a surviving member of the patient's immediate family. If someone other than the patient paid the bill, payment may be made to that person. If the bill has not been paid and the doctor or supplier does not accept assignment, Medical Insurance payment can be made to the person who has a legal obligation to pay the bill for the deceased patient. This person can claim Medical Insurance payment either before or after paying the bill.

G-5. Is there a time limit for submitting a Medicare claim?

A doctor or supplier must submit a claim by December 31 of the following year for services furnished during the first nine months of the year. Claims must be submitted by December 31 of the second following year for services furnished during the last three months of the year.

G-6. Where does a doctor or supplier send Medical Insurance claims?

See Appendix D for the names and addresses of Medicare carriers selected to handle Medical Insurance (Part B) claims in each state.

Each carrier must maintain a toll-free telephone number or numbers so that enrollees may obtain the names, addresses, specialty, and telephone numbers of participating physicians and suppliers. Enrollees may request a copy of an appropriate directory of participating physicians and suppliers. The carrier must mail the directory to the enrollee at no charge.

G-7. Must Medicare claims be paid in a prompt manner?

Carriers and intermediaries must pay Medicare claims promptly. Not less than 95% of "clean claim" payments must be issued, mailed, or otherwise transmitted within specified time limits. A clean claim is a claim that has no defect or impropriety or particular circumstance requiring special treatment that prevents timely payment from being made. The deadline for payment of a clean claim is 30 calendar days.

If payment is not issued, mailed, or otherwise transmitted within 30 calendar days on a clean claim, interest must be paid for the period beginning on the day after the required payment date and ending on the date on which payment is made.

Carriers and intermediaries are prohibited from issuing, mailing or otherwise transmitting payment for any electronic claims within 13 days after their receipt. This prohibition on paying claims is expanded to 26 days for claims not submitted electronically.

APPEALS PROCEDURE

G-8. Does a person have the right to appeal a decision made on a claim?

Yes, if a person disagrees with a decision on the amount Medicare will pay on a claim or whether services received are covered by Medicare, the person has the right to ask for a review of the decision. The notice from Medicare tells the patient the decision made on the claim and what steps to take to appeal the decision. If a person needs more information about the right to appeal, he should contact the local Social Security office, the Medicare intermediary or carrier, or the Quality Improvement Organization (QIO) in his state.

G-9. How does a person appeal a Medical Insurance claim?

After the doctor or supplier submits the claim for payment to the carrier, Medicare will send a notice of the decision made on the claim. If the patient disagrees with the decision, he can ask the Medicare carrier that handled the claim to review it. The patient has six months from the date of the decision to ask the carrier to review it. If the patient disagrees with the carrier's written explanation of its review decision and the amount remaining in question is $100 or more, the patient has six months from the date of the review decision to request a hearing before a carrier hearing officer. The patient may combine claims that have been reviewed or reopened so long as all claims combined are at the proper level of appeal and the appeal for each claim combined is filed on time.

If a person disagrees with the carrier hearing officer's decision and the amount in question is $500 or more, the person has 60 days from the date he receives the decision to request a hearing before an Administrative Law Judge. Cases involving $1,000 or more can eventually be appealed to a federal court.

To determine whether an individual meets the minimum amount in controversy needed for a carrier hearing ($100) or administrative law judge hearing ($500), the following rules apply:

(1) The amount in controversy is computed as the actual amount charged the patient for the items and services in question, less any amount for which payment has been made by the carrier and less any deductible and coinsurance amounts applicable in the particular case.

(2) A single patient may aggregate claims from two or more physicians/suppliers to meet the $100 or $500 thresholds. A single physician/supplier may aggregate claims from two or more patients to meet the $100 or $500 threshold levels of appeal.

(3) Two or more claims may be aggregated by an individual patient to meet the amount in controversy for a carrier hearing only if the claims have previously been reviewed and a request for hearing has been made within six months after the date of the review determination(s).

(4) Two or more claims may be aggregated by an individual patient for an administrative law judge hearing only if the claims have previously been decided by a carrier hearing officer and a request for an administrative law judge hearing has been made within 60 days after receipt of the carrier hearing officer's decision(s).

(5) When requesting a carrier hearing or an administrative law judge hearing, the appellant must specify in the appeal request the specific claims to be aggregated.

Two or more patients may aggregate their claims together to meet the minimum amount in controversy needed for an administrative law judge hearing ($500).

The determination as to whether the amount in controversy is $100 or more is made by the carrier hearing officer. The determination as to whether the amount in controversy is $500 or more is made by the administrative law judge.

When a civil action is filed by either an individual patient or two or more patients, the Centers for Medicare & Medicaid Services may assert that the aggregation principles may be applied to determine the amount in controversy for judicial review ($1,000).

G-10. How does a person request a review by the Medicare carrier that handled the claim?

A reconsideration request must be made in writing and filed at a Social Security Administration or Centers for Medicare & Medicaid Services office, or in the case of a qualified Railroad Retirement beneficiary, filed at a Railroad Retirement Board office. The request must be filed within six months of receipt of the notice of the initial determination, unless an extension of time for filing the request is granted.

The parties to a reconsideration determination are entitled to written notice specifying the reasons for the decision and advising them of their right to a hearing if the amount in question is $100 or more.

G-11. How does a person request a hearing with the carrier hearing officer?

An individual who is dissatisfied with a reconsideration determination is entitled to a hearing if the amount in controversy is $100 or more. The request for a hearing must be made in writing and filed at a Social Security Administration or Centers for Medicare & Medicaid Services office, or in the case of a qualified Railroad Retirement beneficiary, at a Railroad Retirement Board office. The hearing request must be filed within six months after the date of an individual's receipt of notice of the reconsidered determination, unless the deadline is extended.

G-12. How does a person appeal a Hospital Insurance (Part A) decision made by a Quality Improvement Organization (QIO)?

Quality Improvement Organizations (QIOs) make decisions on the need for hospital care. Whenever a patient is admitted to a Medicare-participating hospital, the patient is given *An Important Message From Medicare*, which describes his appeal rights as a hospital patient and supplies the name, address, and phone number of the QIO in his state. The hospital is also required to provide the patient with *How to Request a Review of the Notice of Noncoverage*, which includes a general statement about the post-hospital services to which the patient is entitled.

To determine whether a patient meets the minimum amount in controversy needed for a hearing ($100), the following rules apply:

(1) The amount in controversy is computed as the actual amount charged the patient for the items and services in question, less any amount for which payment has been made by the intermediary and less any deductible and coinsurance amounts applicable in the particular case.

(2) A single patient may aggregate claims from two or more providers to meet the $100 hearing threshold and a single provider may aggregate claims for services provided to one or more patients to meet the $100 hearing threshold.

(3) Two or more claims may be aggregated by an individual patient only if the claims have previously been reconsidered and a request for hearing has been made within 60 days after receipt of the reconsideration determination.

(4) When requesting a hearing, the appellant must specify in the appeal request the specific claims to be aggregated.

Also, two or more patients may aggregate their claims together to meet the minimum amount in controversy needed for a hearing ($100).

The determination as to whether the amount in controversy is $100 or more is made by the administrative law judge.

If a hospital, without consulting the QIO, recommends against admission to the hospital, review of this decision by the QIO may be obtained by writing the QIO requesting a review. If the QIO participated in the preadmission denial, then a reconsideration of the denial can be requested. If an expedited request for review is made within three working days of the denial, the QIO has three working days to respond.

The appeals process for determinations of non-coverage after a patient is admitted to the hospital is similar to the process for pre-admission denials. The hospital cannot charge the patient for the cost of an additional stay unless (1) the hospital or its utilization review committee determines that hospital care is no longer necessary, or the QIO states in writing that hospital care is unnecessary, and (2) the patient receives written notice that charges will be made beginning the third day after receipt of the notice and the decision may be appealed by following procedures specified in the notice.

The hospital must have either the agreement of the physician or the QIO before giving a patient written notice of non-coverage. If the physician, but not the QIO, agrees with the hospital, the patient may make a telephone request to the QIO for review, with a simultaneous written confirmation to the QIO of the request for review. If the patient makes this request prior to noon of the day following receipt of notice of non-coverage, the patient cannot be liable for hospital charges until noon of the working day after receipt of the QIO's decision. The QIO must determine within one full working day of the request (and receipt of pertinent information and/or records from the hospital) the appropriateness of the hospital's decision that the beneficiary no longer requires inpatient hospital care.

If the patient does not appeal, he will be liable for all hospital charges beginning the third day after receipt of the hospital's notice.

If the QIO, rather than the physician, agrees with the hospital's initial notice of non-coverage, the patient can request that the QIO reconsider its decision. If the QIO upholds its initial decision, then the patient is liable for all charges beginning the third day after receipt of the hospital's notice of non-coverage.

The patient should request that the QIO review the hospital's notice of non-coverage as soon as possible. If the patient requests a review while in the hospital or within three days of notice of non-coverage, the QIO must render its decision within three working days.

The patient may request a review by the QIO at any time within 60 days after receipt of the hospital's non-coverage determination. The QIO will have 30 days to issue a decision (unless the request was made within three days of receipt of the non-coverage determination or while the patient was hospitalized).

If the HMO, rather than the hospital, makes the determination of non-coverage, the patient may request an immediate QIO review of the determination.

For the immediate QIO review process, the following rules apply: (1) the patient or authorized representative must submit the request for immediate review to the QIO that has an agreement with the hospital in writing or by telephone by noon of the first working day after receipt of the written notice of the determination that the hospital stay is no longer necessary, (2) on the date it receives the patient's request, the QIO must notify the HMO that a request for immediate review has been filed, (3) the HMO must supply any information that the QIO requires to conduct its review by the close of business of the first full working day immediately following the day the enrollee submits the request for review, (4) in response to a request from the HMO, the hospital must submit medical records to the QIO by close of business of the first full working day immediately following the day the HMO makes its request, (5) the QIO must solicit views of the patient who requested the immediate QIO review, and (6) the QIO must make a determination and notify the patient, the hospital, and the HMO by close of business of the first working day after it receives the information from the hospital, the HMO, or both.

The HMO continues to be financially responsible for the costs of the hospital stay until noon of the calendar day following the day the QIO notifies the patient of its review determination. However, the hospital may not charge the HMO if it was the hospital (acting on behalf of the patient) that filed the request for an immediate QIO review, and the QIO upholds the non-coverage determination made by the HMO.

The patient may appeal a QIO reconsideration decision to an Administrative Law Judge within 60 days, provided the amount of the controversy is at least $200. Cases involving $2,000 or more can eventually be appealed to a federal court.

G-13. How does a person appeal all other Hospital Insurance (Part A) claims?

Appeals of decisions on all other services covered under Hospital Insurance (skilled nursing facility care, home health care, hospice services, and some inpatient hospital matters not handled by QIOs) are handled by Medicare intermediaries. If a patient disagrees with the intermediary's initial decision, he may request a reconsideration. The request can be submitted directly to the intermediary or through a Social Security office. Any Social Security office will help the patient request a reconsideration.

If a patient disagrees with the intermediary's reconsideration decision and the amount in question is $100 or more, the patient has 60 days from the date he received the reconsideration decision to request a hearing by an Administrative Law Judge. Cases involving $1,000 or more can eventually be appealed to a federal court.

G-14. How does a person appeal a decision made by a Health Maintenance Organization (HMO)?

If a person has Medicare coverage through an HMO, decisions about coverage and payment for services will usually be made by the HMO. When the HMO makes a decision to deny payment for Medicare-covered services or refuses to provide Medicare-covered supplies requested by the patient, the patient will be given a *Notice of Initial Determination*. The HMO is also required to provide a full, written explanation of the patient's appeal rights.

If a patient believes that the decision of the HMO was not correct, the patient has the right to ask for a reconsideration. The patient must file a request for reconsideration within 60 days after the patient receives the *Notice of Initial Determination*. The request for reconsideration may be mailed or delivered to the HMO or to a Social Security office.

The HMO must reconsider its initial determination to deny payments or services. If the HMO does not rule fully in the patient's favor, the HMO must send the patient's reconsideration request and its reconsideration determination to the Centers for Medicare & Medicaid Services for a review and determination.

A patient may not proceed to the next level of administrative review until the HMO issues its decision or refers the matter to the Centers for Medicare & Medicaid Services.

An HMO must act on the patient's reconsideration request within 60 calendar days from the date of receipt of the request. If the reconsideration determination made by the HMO is entirely favorable to the patient, the HMO must notify the patient within the 60-calendar-day period. If the HMO cannot make a decision that is fully favorable to the patient, the organization must submit the case file to the Centers for Medicare & Medicaid Services within the 60-calendar-day period.

For good cause, the Centers for Medicare & Medicaid Services may allow exceptions to the 60-day limit. Good cause is defined as unusual circumstances such as natural disasters which make it difficult or impossible for the patient to provide necessary information in a timely way. Failure of the HMO to provide the patient with a reconsideration determination within the 60-day limit or to obtain a good cause extension constitutes an adverse determination.

If the patient disagrees with the decision of the Centers for Medicare & Medicaid Services, and the amount in question is $100 or more, the patient has 60 days from receipt of the decision to request a hearing before an Administrative Law Judge. The amount in question can include any combination of Hospital Insurance and Medical Insurance services. Cases involving $1,000 or more can eventually be appealed to a federal court.

The rules regarding an immediate QIO review of a determination of noncoverage of inpatient hospital care by an HMO or hospital are discussed at G-12.

G-15. What happens if an organization providing items or services to a person under Medicare ceases to continue providing those items or services?

An organization must provide assurances to the Centers for Medicare & Medicaid Services that in the event it ceases to provide items or services, the organization will provide or arrange for supplemental coverage of benefits related to a pre-existing condition. This coverage must be provided to individuals enrolled with the organization who receive Medicare benefits and must continue for the lesser of six months or the duration of the contract period.

MEDICAID

OVERVIEW

H-1. What is Medicaid?

Title XIX of the *Social Security Act* is a federal-state matching entitlement program that pays for medical assistance for certain vulnerable and needy individuals and families with low incomes and resources. The program, known as Medicaid, became law in 1965 as a jointly funded cooperative venture between the federal and state governments to assist states furnishing medical assistance to eligible needy persons. Medicaid is the largest program funding medical and health-related services for America's poorest people.

The Social Security Act authorizes grants to states for Medicaid to certain individuals whose income and resources are insufficient to meet the cost of necessary medical care. The Medicaid program is jointly financed by the federal and state governments and administered by the states. Within federal rules, each state chooses eligible groups, types and ranges of services, payment levels for most services, and administrative and operating procedures. The nature and scope of a state's Medicaid program is described in the state plan that the state submits to the Centers for Medicare & Medicaid Services for approval. The plan is amended whenever necessary to reflect changes in federal or state law, changes in policy, or court decisions.

Federal responsibility for the Medicaid program lies with the Centers for Medicare & Medicaid Services in the Department of Health and Human Services.

States are required to provide certain basic medical assistance services to eligible recipients. These mandatory Medicaid services include inpatient and outpatient hospital care, health screening, diagnosis and treatment to children, family planning, physician services and nursing facility services to individuals over age 21. States may also elect to cover any of over 30 specified optional services, which include prescription drugs, clinic services, personal care services, and services provided in intermediate care facilities for the mentally retarded.

To qualify for Medicaid, applicants must have both incomes and assets below certain limits, which vary from state to state.

Within broad national guidelines established by federal statutes, regulations and policies, each of the states (1) establishes its own eligibility standards, (2) determines the type, amount, duration, and scope of services, (3) sets the rate of payment for services, and (4) administers its own program. Medicaid policies for eligibility and services are complex, and vary considerably even among similar-sized and/or adjacent states. Thus, a person who is eligible for Medicaid in one state might not be eligible in another state; and the services provided by one state may differ considerably in amount, duration, or scope from the services provided in a similar or neighboring state. In addition, Medicaid eligibility and/or services within a state can change during the year.

Medicaid serves as a supplement to health insurance coverage provided by Medicare. Medicaid pays for extended nursing home care for elderly people who cannot afford to pay for it themselves. For those who qualify, Medicaid pays Medicare premiums, as well as Medicare coinsurance and deductibles. It may even pay the full cost of some services not covered by Medicare.

Nursing home care is the largest catastrophic health care expense for the elderly. According to the American Association of Retired Persons, the average annual cost of nursing home care exceeds $50,000. Many elderly persons enter nursing homes and deplete their life savings until they are impoverished. Once impoverished, they qualify for Medicaid coverage.

Many attorneys and financial planners provide counsel to their upper and middle-class elderly clients on how to protect their wealth and still qualify for Medicaid. Many elderly persons who are not in poverty have found ways to get Medicaid to pay for nursing home care. But changes made by the *Omnibus Budget Reconciliation Act of 1993* and the *Deficit Reduction Act of 2005* make it much more difficult for upper and middle-class persons to qualify for Medicaid.

H-2. What portion of Medicaid expenses are paid by the federal government?

The federal government pays a proportion of the medical assistance expenditures under each state's Medicaid program, known as the Federal Medical Assistance Percentage (FMAP). The FMAP is determined annually by a formula that compares the state's average per capita income level with the national income average. States with a higher per capita income level are reimbursed a smaller share of their costs. By law, the FMAP cannot be lower than 50% nor higher than 83%. In fiscal 2007, the FMAPs vary from 50% (to 12 states) to 75.89% (to Mississippi).

In addition, the *Deficit Reduction Act of 2005* included temporary FMAP adjustments for states affected by Hurricane Katrina and for the State of Alaska (preventing Alaska's FMAP from dropping below 2005's level in 2006 or 2007).

The federal government reimburses states for 100% of the cost of services provided through facilities of the Indian Health Service. The federal government also shares in each state's expenditures for the administration of the Medicaid program. Most administrative costs are matched at 50% for all states, with higher rates for certain activities such as development of mechanized claims processing systems. The Medicaid statute does provide for higher matching rates for certain functions and activities.

Federal payments to states for medical assistance have no set limit (cap); rather, the federal government matches (at FMAP rates) state expenditures for the mandatory services plus the optional services that the individual state decides to cover for eligible recipients, and matches (at the appropriate administrative rate) necessary and proper administrative costs.

MEDICAID ELIGIBILITY

H-3. What major groups are states required to cover?

States have some discretion in determining who their Medicaid programs will cover and the financial criteria for Medicaid eligibility. To be eligible for federal funds, states are required to provide Medicaid coverage for most individuals who receive federally assisted income maintenance payments, as well as for related groups not receiving cash payments. Examples of the mandatory Medicaid eligibility groups include the following:

- Individuals who meet the requirements of Aid to Families with Dependent Children (AFDC) that were in effect in their state on July 16, 1996.

- Supplemental Security Income (SSI) recipients (or in states using more restrictive criteria–aged, blind and disabled individuals who meet criteria which are more restrictive than those of the SSI program and which were in place in the state's approved Medicaid plan as of January 1, 1972).

- Infants born to Medicaid-eligible pregnant women. Medicaid eligibility must continue throughout the first year of life so long as the infant remains in the mother's household and she remains eligible, or would be eligible if she were still pregnant.

- Children under age 6 and pregnant women who meet the state's AFDC financial requirements or whose family income is at or below 133% of the federal poverty level. (The minimum mandatory income level for pregnant women and infants in certain states may be higher than 133%, if as of certain dates the states had established a higher percentage for covering these groups.) States are required to extend Medicaid eligibility until age 19 to all children in families with incomes at or below the federal poverty level. Once eligibility is established, pregnant women remain eligible for Medicaid through the end of the calendar month ending 60 days after the end of the pregnancy regardless of any change in family income. States are not required to have a resource test for these poverty level related groups. However, any resource test imposed can be no more restrictive than that of the AFDC program for infants and children and the SSI program for pregnant women.

- Recipients of adoption assistance and foster care under the Social Security Act.

- Certain Medicare beneficiaries. (See H-11.)

- Special protected groups who lose cash assistance because of the cash programs' rules, but who may keep Medicaid for a period of time. Examples are: persons who lose AFDC or SSI payments due to earnings from work or increased Social Security benefits; and two-parent, unemployed families whose AFDC cash assistance time is limited by the state and who are provided a full 12 months of Medicaid coverage following termination of cash assistance.

Certain qualified aliens, including certain permanent residents, certain asylees, certain refugees, certain aliens whose deportation has been withheld, and certain veterans and their spouses and dependents, are covered under Medicaid. (Asylees, refugees, and deportees are only required to be covered by Medicaid for the first five years of their status in those categories.)

H-4. What are "SSI States"?

States have two options with regard to coverage of SSI recipients. In most states (SSI States) the Medicaid program includes all SSI recipients. Other states, however, cover only those persons who are age 65, disabled, or blind and who meet a means test that is more restrictive than the SSI means test. These states are called "Section 209(b) states." For example, a Section 209(b) state may define disability more narrowly than the federal definition for SSI entitlement.

H-5. Do states have the option of providing additional Medicaid coverage?

Yes, states have the option of providing Medicaid coverage for "categorically needy" groups. These optional groups share characteristics of the mandatory groups, but the eligibility criteria are somewhat more liberally defined. Examples of the optional groups that states may cover as categorically needy (and for which they will receive federal matching funds) under the Medicaid program include the following:

- Infants up to age one and pregnant women not covered under the mandatory rules whose family income is below 185% of the federal poverty level (the percentage is set by each state).

- Certain aged, blind, or disabled adults who have incomes above those requiring mandatory coverage, but below the federal poverty level.

- Children under age 21 who meet what were the AFDC income and resource requirements in effect in their state on July 16, 1996 (even though they do not meet the mandatory eligibility requirements).

- Children under age 19, or a younger age specified by the state, in households with incomes at or below 100% of the federal poverty level. States may provide a full, continuous 12 months of eligibility for such children.

- Institutionalized individuals with incomes and resources below specified limits. The amount is set by each state–up to 300% of the SSI federal benefits rate.

- Persons who would be eligible if institutionalized but are receiving care under home and community-based services waivers.

- Recipients of state supplementary income payments.

- TB-infected persons who would be financially eligible for Medicaid at the SSI income level (only for TB-related ambulatory services and TB drugs).

- "Medically needy" persons (described below).

The option to have a "Medically Needy" program allows states to extend Medicaid eligibility to additional qualified persons who may have too much income to qualify under the mandatory or optional categorically needy groups. This option allows them to "spend down" to Medicaid eligibility by incurring medical and/or remedial care expenses to offset their excess income, thereby reducing it to a level below the maximum allowed by that state's Medicaid plan. States may also allow families to establish eligibility as medically needy by paying monthly premiums to the state in an amount equal to the difference between family income (reduced by unpaid expenses, if any, incurred for medical care in previous months) and the income eligibility standard.

Eligibility for the medically needy program does not need to be as extensive as the categorically needy program. But states that elect to include the medically needy under their plans are required to include certain children under age 18 and pregnant women who except for income and resources would be eligible as categorically needy. They may choose to provide coverage to other medically needy persons: aged, blind, and/or disabled persons; certain relatives of children deprived of parental support and care; and certain other financially eligible children up to age 21.

States can expand Medicaid eligibility for children under the State Children's Health Insurance Program. In order to be eligible for federal funds, states must submit to, and obtain approval from, the Secretary for Health and Human Services for a State Child Health Plan. States that elect to use the child health assistance funds to expand Medicaid eligibility and meet conditions for participating in the program are eligible to receive an enhanced Medicaid match for "optional targeted low-income children." The enhanced Medicaid match is the state's current Federal Medical Assistance Percentage (FMAP) increased by 30% of the difference between 100% and the current FMAP. "Optional targeted low-income children" are defined as targeted low-income children who would not qualify for Medicaid based on the plan that was in effect on April 15, 1997. It would not apply to expenditures for children below the federal poverty level who were born after September 30, 1983.

Coverage may start retroactive to any or all of the three months prior to application if the person would have been eligible during the retroactive period. Coverage generally stops at the end of the month in which a person's circumstances change. Most states have additional "states only" programs to provide medical assistance to specified poor persons who do not qualify for Medicaid. Federal funds are not provided for state-only programs.

Medicaid does not provide health care services for all poor persons. To be eligible for Medicaid, a person must belong to one of the designated groups listed above, as well as meet income and assets/resources tests. Even under the broadest provisions of federal law (except for a few emergency services for certain persons), the Medicaid program does not provide health care services, even for very poor persons, unless they are under age 21, pregnant, aged, blind, disabled, or in certain AFDC-type families.

MEDICAID SERVICES

H-6. What basic services must be offered by Medicaid?

The Social Security Act requires that a state Medicaid program must offer medical assistance for certain basic services to most categorically needy populations. These services generally include the following:

- Inpatient hospital services.

- Outpatient hospital services.

- Prenatal care.

- Vaccines for children.

- Physician services.

- Nursing facility services for persons aged 21 or older.

- Family planning services and supplies.

- Rural health clinic services.

- Home health care for persons eligible for skilled nursing services.

- Laboratory and x-ray services.

- Pediatric and family nurse practitioner services.

- Nurse-midwife services.

- Federally-qualified health-center (FQHC) services, and ambulatory services of an FQHC that would be available in other settings.

- Early and periodic screening, diagnostic, and treatment (EPSDT) services for children under age 21.

If a state chooses to include the medically needy population, the state plan must provide, as a minimum, the following services:

- Prenatal care and delivery services for pregnant women.

- Ambulatory services to individuals under age 18 and individuals entitled to institutional services.

- Home health services to individuals entitled to nursing facility services.

States may also receive federal matching funds for providing certain optional services.

The most common optional Medicaid services include:

- Home health care services (eligibility does not depend on a need or discharge from a skilled nursing facility).

- Diagnostic services.

- Clinic services.

- Intermediate care facilities for the mentally retarded.

- Prescribed drugs and prosthetic devices.

- Optometrist services and eyeglasses.

- Dental care.

- Hearing aids.

- Nursing facility services for children under age 21.

- Transportation services.

- Rehabilitation and physical therapy services.

- Home and community-based care to certain persons with chronic impairments (this one is an option with an approved waiver).

H-7. Is AIDS covered under Medicaid?

Serving at least 50% of all persons living with AIDS and up to 90% of all children with AIDS, Medicaid is the largest single payer of direct medical services for persons with AIDS.

States must provide the full range of Medicaid services covered in the state plan to eligible persons with HIV disease, and they may also provide optional services that are often appropriate for people with HIV/AIDS, such as targeted case management, preventive services, and hospice care. All states cover FDA-approved prescribed drugs.

Most adults with AIDs or HIV-related illnesses who qualify for Medicaid do so because they are disabled, have low income, and limited assets. Others in families with dependent children may become eligible for Medicaid by meeting certain income and resource standards. Still others who may have too much income or resources may become Medicaid eligible based on their medical expenses. Individuals should contact their state Medicaid agency for state-specific criteria.

H-8. What optional services may a state elect to provide?

States may elect to provide a number of other services for which federal matching funds are available. Some of the most frequently covered optional services are: clinic services, medical transportation services, intermediate care facility services for the mentally re-tarded, optometrist services and eyeglasses, prescribed drugs, case management services, prosthetic devices, dental services, physical therapy, occupational therapy, speech therapy, hospice care, respiratory care services, personal care services furnished in a home, and at the state's option, in another location, and home and community-based care for func-tionally disabled elderly persons.

PAYMENT UNDER MEDICAID

H-9. How are providers of health care services paid under Medicaid?

Medicaid operates as a vendor payment program, with states paying providers directly. Providers participating in Medicaid must accept Medicaid payment rates as payment in full. States may pay for Medicaid services through various prepayment arrangements, such as health maintenance organizations (HMOs). Within federally-imposed upper limits and specific restrictions, each state generally has broad discretion in determining the payment methodology and payment rate for services. Generally, payment rates must be sufficient to enlist enough providers so that covered services are available at least to the extent that comparable care and services are available to the general population within that geographic area. States must make additional payments to qualified hospitals that provide inpatient services to a disproportionate number of Medicaid recipients and/or to other low-income persons under what is known as the "disproportionate share hospital" (DSH) adjustment. These payments are limited.

States may impose nominal deductibles, coinsurance or co-payments on some Medicaid recipients for certain services. However, certain Medicaid recipients must be excluded from cost sharing: pregnant women, children under age 18, hospital or nursing home patients who are expected to contribute most of their income to institutional care, and categorically needy recipients enrolled in HMOs. In addition, emergency services and family planning services must be exempt from co-payments for all recipients.

The federal government pays a proportion of the medical assistance expenditures under each states Medicaid program, known as the Federal Medical Assistance Percent-age (FMAP). The FMAP is determined annually by a formula that compares the state's average per capita income level with the national income average. States with a higher per capita income level are reimbursed a smaller share of their costs. By law, the FMAP cannot be lower than 50% nor higher than 83%. (See H-2.)

H-10. What is the amount and duration of Medicaid services?

Within broad federal guidelines, states determine the duration and amount of services offered under their Medicaid programs. They may limit, for example, the number of days of hospital care or the number of physician visits covered. But some restrictions apply: Limits must result in a sufficient level of services to reasonably achieve the purpose of the benefits. Limits on required (non-optional) benefits may not discriminate among beneficiaries based on medical diagnosis or condition.

In general, states are required to provide Medicaid coverage for comparable amounts, duration, and scope of services to all categorically-needy and categorically-related eligible persons. There are two important exceptions: (1) Medically necessary health care services identified under the early and periodic screening, diagnostic, and treatment (EPSDT) program for eligible children that are within the scope of mandatory or optional services under federal law must be covered even if those services are not included as part of the covered services in that state's plan (i.e., only these specific children might receive that specific service), and (2) States may require "waivers" to pay for otherwise-uncovered home and community-based services (HCBS) for Medicaid-eligible persons who might otherwise be institutionalized (i.e., only persons so designated might receive HCBS). States have few limitations on the services that may be covered under these waivers as long as the services are cost effective (except that, other than as a part of respite care, they may not provide room and board for recipients). With certain exceptions, a state's Medicaid plan must allow recipients to have freedom of choice among participating providers of health care.

H-11. How does Medicaid help with Medicare coverage for the needy, elderly, and disabled?

Persons who are qualified for Medicare and who are poor may also receive help from Medicaid. For persons who are eligible for *full* Medicaid coverage, the Medicare health care coverage is supplemented by services that are available under their state's Medicaid program. As each state elects, services such as prescription drugs, eyeglasses, hearing aids, and nursing facility care beyond the 100 day limit covered by Medicare may be provided by the Medicaid program. However, if a person is a Medicare beneficiary, payments for any services covered by Medicare are made by Medicare before any payments are made by the Medicaid program; Medicaid is always "payor of last resort."

In addition, there are three groups of Medicare beneficiaries who may not be fully eligible for Medicaid, but who do receive some help through their state Medicaid program. Most of the Medicare beneficiaries helped by Medicaid are those identified as (1) Qualified Medicare Beneficiaries (QMBs) and as (2) Specified Low-Income Medicare Beneficiaries (SLMBs). QMBs are those Medicare beneficiaries who have resources at or below twice the standard allowed under the SSI program, and incomes below 100% of the federal poverty level. This includes people who are also fully eligible for Medicaid. For QMBs, the state pays the Hospital Insurance (Part A) and Medical Insurance (Part B) premiums and Medicare coinsurance and deductibles, subject to limits that states may impose on payment rates. SLMBs are Medicare beneficiaries with resources like the QMBs, yet with incomes that are higher–but still less than 120% of the federal poverty level. For SLMBs, the Medicaid program pays the Medical Insurance premiums. Persons who previously qualified for Medicare because of disability, but who lost entitlement because of their return to work (despite the disability), are allowed to purchase Medicare Hospital Insurance and Medical Insurance coverage. Medicaid assists a few persons known as Qualified Disabled and Working Individuals (QDWIs) who have incomes below 200% of the federal poverty level, but who do not meet any other Medicaid assistance category. These QDWIs have their Hospital Insurance (Part A) premium (and sometimes all or part of their Medical Insurance (Part B) premium) paid by the Medicaid program in their states.

Medicaid pays Medical Insurance premiums for SLMBs with incomes up to 135% of the federal poverty level. States must permit all who qualify to apply. However, states must limit the number selected in a calendar year so that the aggregate cost for the number served is estimated to equal the state's allocation from the federal government in that year. Selection by states is on a first-come, first-served basis.

LONG-TERM CARE

H-12. Does Medicaid provide coverage for long-term care?

The greatest change from the original Medicaid program has been the growth of Medicaid's substantial role in long-term care. Almost 45% of care for people using nursing facilities or home health services in the United States in recent years is paid for by the Medicaid program. But a much larger percentage is paid for by Medicaid for those persons who use more than four months of such long-term health care. Data for 2002 show that Medicaid payments for nursing facility and home health care totaled about $82 billion for more than 7.3 million recipients of these services—an average expenditure of about $11,250 per long-term care recipient. $57 billion of the total was spent on only 1.8 million residents of nursing facilities–an average of over $31,500 per recipient.

EXEMPT INCOME AND RESOURCES

H-13. Are certain income and resources exempt from the financial eligibility standards that govern Medicaid eligibility?

A single individual will not qualify for Medicaid in most states unless he has less than $2,000 in countable assets.

In determining whether applicants for Medicaid meet asset criteria, certain assets are considered "countable" and other assets are considered "exempt." Exempt assets include the following:

- The cash value of permanent life insurance policies up to $1,500 of face value, and all life insurance policies with no cash value (term insurance).

- Household furnishings (furniture, paintings, appliances, etc.), which are exempt only while used in the applicant's home.

- Burial funds up to $1,500 (reduced by the face value of any cash value life insurance polices otherwise exempted and any amounts held in an irrevocable burial fund trust). There is no dollar limit if the burial plan is irrevocable.

- Property used in a trade or business.

- Burial space (grave site, crypt, mausoleum, urn, grave marker).

- One automobile of any value: (1) for a married couple where one spouse is institutionalized, (2) if equipped for a handicapped person, (3) if used to obtain medical treatment, or (4) if used for employment. This exemption is limited to $4,500 in all other cases.

- Up to $500,000 of equity in a home, provided it is the person's principal place of residence. This includes the land on which the home sits and any adjoining property. States may choose to increase this amount up to $750,000.

- Property owned with one or more other individuals if the other owners use the property as the principal place of residence and would be forced to move if the property were sold.

- Personal effects, including clothing, photographs, jewelry, etc.

The home is treated as a resource after the individual has been institutionalized for six months, unless the individual's spouse or minor, disabled or blind child continues to reside in the home, or it can be shown that the individual may be able to leave the institution and return home.

Exempt assets lose that status upon the death of the Medicaid recipient. Therefore, the state may claim reimbursement from the recipient's estate. Medicaid authorities are sometimes granted a lien against the home, collectible after the death of the recipient (or the death of certain relatives living in the home) to compensate for Medicaid benefits paid to the homeowner.

Medicaid applicants must also meet income tests that vary by state. In some of the states, there is no upper income limit for persons in nursing homes. The remaining states have "income caps" in determining eligibility for nursing home coverage. If a person has income below the private cost of nursing home care in one of the states where there is no upper income limit, he meets Medicaid's income test. For example, if a man has monthly income of $2,500 and the private cost of nursing home care is $3,000 (and he has less than $2,000 in countable assets), he will qualify for Medicaid. He will be required to pay all of his income, except for a small "personal needs allowance," to the nursing home and Medicaid pays the balance of the bill.

Federal law requires states with "income caps" to set their "income caps" no higher than 300% of the Federal SSI benefit level ($623 in 2007). Thus, the "income cap" can be no greater than $1,869 in 2006. Not all of the states using "income caps" set their cap at the maximum allowable level (300% of the SSI benefit level). For example, if a person's monthly income is $1,550 in a state that sets its cap at $1,500, he does not qualify for Medicaid.

SPOUSAL IMPOVERISHMENT

H-14. Are there guidelines regarding the amount of income the community spouse of a nursing home resident can maintain?

The expense of nursing home care—which can range from $2,000 to $5,000 a month or more—can rapidly deplete the lifetime savings of elderly couples. The Medicare Catastrophic Coverage Act of 1988 mandated special Medicaid eligibility rules for couples when one member needs nursing home care. The rules protect income and resources for the other member of the couple. These rules are known as the spousal impoverishment rules. They apply in all 50 states and the District of Columbia.

H-15. What are the resource eligibility requirements?

The spousal impoverishment provisions apply where the member of the couple who is in a nursing facility or medical institution is expected to remain there for at least 30 days. When the couple applies for Medicaid, an assessment of their resources is conducted. The couple's resources are combined and exemptions for the home, household goods, an automobile, and burial funds are taken into account. (See H-13.) The result is the spousal resource amount. The spousal resource amount is the state's minimum resource standard ($20,328 in 2007); or the spousal share, which is equal to one-half of the couple's combined resources, not to exceed the maximum permitted by the state ($101,640 in 2007).

In order to determine whether the spouse residing in a medical facility is eligible for Medicaid, a determination of the couple's total countable resources must be made. All resources held by both spouses are considered to be available to the spouse in the medical facility, except for the protected resource amount (PRA). This PRA is the greatest of:

- The spousal resource amount.

- The state spousal resource standard, which is the amount that the state has determined will be protected for the community spouse.

- An amount transferred to the community spouse for her/his support as directed by a court order.

- An amount designated by a state hearing officer to raise the community spouse's protected resources up to the minimum monthly maintenance needs standard (150% of the federal poverty level for a household of two).

The remainder becomes attributable to the spouse that is residing in a medical institution as countable resources. If the amount of resources is below the state's resource standard, the individual is eligible for Medicaid. Once resource eligibility is determined, resources of the community spouse are not attributed to the spouse in the medical facility.

H-16. What are the income eligibility requirements?

The community spouse's income is not considered available to the spouse who is in the medical facility, and the two individuals are not considered a couple for these purposes. The state must use the income eligibility standards for one person rather than two. Therefore, the standard income eligibility process for Medicaid is used. (See H-13.)

H-17. What is the process for the post-eligibility treatment of income?

This process is followed after an individual in a nursing facility/medical institution is determined to be eligible for Medicaid. The post-eligibility process is used to determine how much the spouse in the medical facility must contribute toward the cost of nursing facility/institutional care. The process also determines how much of the income of the spouse who is in the medical facility is actually protected for use by the community spouse.

Deductions are made from the total income of the spouse who is residing in the medical facility in the following order:

- A personal needs allowance of at least $40 ($30 for individuals on SSI).

- The community spouse's monthly income allowance—between $1,650 (from July 1, 2006 through June 30, 2007) and $2,541 (in 2007)—as long as the income is actually made available to the spouse.

- A family monthly income allowance.

- An amount for medical expenses incurred by the spouse who is in the medical facility.

The sum of these deductions subtracted from the income of the individual who is in the medical facility will result in the amount the individual must contribute to the cost of care.

MEDICAID TRANSFER RULES

H-18. Can a person transfer property in order to meet the eligibility requirements for Medicaid?

Transfers of property for less than fair market value prior to applying for Medicaid benefits can result in a denial of benefits. States may delay eligibility for Medicaid benefits for a period of time whenever it is determined that a person institutionalized in a medical institution or nursing facility has disposed of resources for less than fair market value within 60 months before application for Medicaid benefits. (The look-back period is 36 months for transfers made prior to February 8, 2006, the effective date of the *Deficit Reduction Act of 2005* (DRA).) A transfer is an outright gift, or an exchange for something worth less than the full value of the transferred property. For example, if a person owns an antique car valued at $50,000, and sells it to his son for $1,000, he has made an improper transfer of $49,000.

Certain transfers can be made within 60 months of the application without loss of Medicaid eligibility. The family home may be transferred to (1) the community spouse (noninstitutionalized spouse), (2) a child who is under age 21, blind, or permanently and totally disabled, (3) an adult son or daughter residing in the home and providing care that delayed the person's need for care in a medical institution or nursing facility for at least two years, (4) a trust created solely for the benefit of disabled children of the applicant, (5) certain trusts created for a disabled child or grandchild under age 65, and (6) a brother or sister who has an ownership interest in the house and who has been living in the home for at least one year immediately before the person's admission for care.

Also, eligibility is unaffected if the transferor can prove that the intent of the transfer was to dispose of the resources either at fair market value or for other valuable consideration, or the exclusive purpose of the transfer was not to qualify for Medicaid. States can also grant eligibility where denial would amount to undue hardship.

All transfers of jointly-owned property to others are deemed to the Medicaid applicant. This penalty applies when the action taken by a co-owner reduces or eliminates the Medicaid applicant's ownership or control of the asset.

Two ways to transfer assets to family members without disqualifying for Medicaid benefits are (1) by transferring the assets to family members more than 60 months before the person applies for Medicaid benefits, and (2) if the applicant is already in a nursing home or about to go into one, by retaining enough assets to pay for 60 months of care, transferring the balance, and not applying for Medicaid until 60 months after the date on which the last asset transfer is completed.

A controversial federal law purports to subject a person to criminal penalties if each of the following occurs: (1) the person counsels or assists another to transfer assets, (2) the person charges a fee for this service, (3) the assets are transferred, (4) the transfer is made in an effort to become eligible for Medicaid, and (5) a period of ineligibility for Medicaid is the result of the transfer of assets. The U.S. Department of Justice has indicated it will not enforce this criminal provision and, in addition, has been enjoined by a federal district court from enforcing it.

H-19. How is the penalty period determined after an improper transfer of assets?

Under the *Deficit Reduction Act of 2005* (DRA), the penalty period of ineligibility for an improper transfer—see H-18—begins on the later of the first day of the month of the transfer or "the date on which the individual is eligible for medical assistance under the State plan…based on an approved application for such care but for the application of the penalty period." The penalty lasts for the number of months equal to the total value of transferred property divided by the average cost of nursing home care to a private patient in the state or community of the applicant. All transfers made in the 60 months prior to the application date are aggregated in determining the length of the penalty period. There is no limit to the length of the penalty period.

For example, a Medicaid applicant who improperly transfers a house worth $350,000 in a state with an average cost of nursing home care of $3,500 a month will be penalized with 100 months of ineligibility for Medicaid ($350,000 ÷ $3,500 = 100). But if a person gives away a house worth $350,000 and then waits more than 60 months to apply for Medicaid, he or she does not have to report the transfer and will not incur the period of ineligibility.

Transfers made prior to February 8, 2006, the effective date of the DRA, are considered separately; and the period of ineligibility for each generally began either the month in which the resources were transferred or the month following the transfer, depending on the rules of the state.

If both spouses enter a nursing home at or near the same time, states are required to apportion the penalty between the spouses so that only one penalty applies. For example, an improper transfer of $70,000 in a state with a nursing home cost of $3,500 will cause each spouse to be ineligible for 10 months ($70,000 ÷ $3,500 = 20 ÷ 2 = 10).

A Medicaid applicant cannot have a portion of the transferred property returned to eliminate the transfer penalty. All assets transferred for less than fair market value must be returned in order to eliminate some or all of the penalty period.

Each state has procedures for waiver of the transfer penalty when the transfer penalty results in undue hardship.

H-20. What are the rules under Medicaid regarding the purchase of annuities?

Under the *Deficit Reduction Act of 2005* (DRA), purchasing an annuity by or on behalf of an applicant is considered an improper transfer of assets—see H-18 and H-19—unless the annuity meets certain requirements.

The purchase of an annuity will not be treated as an improper transfer of assets if

1. the state is named as the primary remainder beneficiary for at least the total amount of medical assistance paid by Medicaid on behalf of the applicant;

2. the state is named as the secondary beneficiary after the community spouse or minor or disabled child;

3. the annuity is purchased inside or with proceeds from a retirement account (IRA, Roth IRA, SEP-IRA, etc.)

Any annuity purchased on behalf of a Medicaid applicant must be irrevocable, nonassignable, actuarially sound, and provide for payments in equal amounts during the term of the annuity, with no deferral and no balloon payments.

Annuities purchased prior to February 8, 2006, the effective date of the DRA, are governed by state-specific provisions. At a minimum, pre-DRA annuities must be actuarially sound, not paying out over a time period exceeding the life expectancy of the Medicaid applicant.

TRUSTS

H-21. Can a trust be used to shelter a Medicaid applicant's assets?

There are considerable limits on the use of trusts to shelter a Medicaid applicant's assets. Trust assets created or funded by a Medicaid applicant or by his or her spouse are considered available to the applicant to the extent the applicant derives any benefit from the trust.

If an institutionalized person or spouse (or, at the option of a state, a noninstitutionalized person or spouse) disposes of trust assets for less than fair market value on or after the *look-back date* for trusts, the person is ineligible for Medicaid for the following time period:

- For an institutionalized person, the number of months of ineligibility is equal to the total of all assets transferred on or after the look-back date divided by the average monthly cost to a private patient of nursing facility services in the state at the time of application. Ineligibility begins on the first day of the first month during or after which assets have been transferred for less than fair market value.

- For a noninstitutionalized person, the number of months of ineligibility may not be greater than a number equal to the total value of all assets transferred on or after the look-back date, divided by the average monthly cost to a private patient of nursing facility services in the state at the time of application. Ineligibility begins on the first day of the first month during or after which assets have been transferred for less than fair market value.

The *look-back period* in the case of payments from a trust or portions of a trust that are treated as assets disposed of is 60 months before (1) the first date on which an institutionalized person is both institutionalized and has applied for Medicaid, or (2) the first date on which a noninstitutionalized person applies for Medicaid, or, if later, the date on which the individual disposes of assets for less than fair market value.

An individual is considered to have established a trust if assets of the individual were used to form all or part of the corpus of the trust and any of the following individuals established the trust other than by will:

- The individual.

- The individual's spouse.

- A person, including a court or administrative body, with legal authority to act in place of or on behalf of the individual or the individual's spouse.

- A person, including any court or administrative body, acting at the direction or upon the request of the individual or the individual's spouse.

In the case of a revocable trust, (1) the corpus of the trust is considered a resource available to the individual, (2) payments from the trust to or for the benefit of the individual are considered income of the individual, and (3) any other payments from the trust are considered assets disposed of by the individual.

Assets are defined as all income and resources of the individual and the individual's spouse, including any income or resources which the individual or the individual's spouse is entitled to but does not receive because of action: (1) by the individual or the individual's spouse, (2) by a person, including a court or administrative body, with legal authority to act in place of or on behalf of the individual or the individual's spouse, or (3) by any person, including any court or administrative body, acting at the direction or upon the request of the individual or the individual's spouse.

In the case of an irrevocable trust:

- If there are any circumstances under which payment from the trust could be made to or for the benefit of the individual, the portion of the corpus from which, or the income on the corpus from which, payment to the individual could be made is considered resources available to the individual, and payments from that portion of the corpus or income: (1) to or from the benefit of the individual, is considered income of the individual, and (2) for any other purpose, is considered a transfer of assets by the individual. (See definition of "asset" above.)

- Any portion of the trust from which, or any income on the corpus from which, no payment could under any circumstances be made to the individual, is considered, as of the date of establishment of the trust (or, if later, the date on which payment to the individual was foreclosed) to be assets disposed of by the individual, and the value of the trust is determined by including the amount of any payments made from such portion of the trust after that date.

A trust includes any legal instrument or device that is similar to a trust but includes an annuity only to such extent and in such manner as the Department of Health and Human Services specifies.

H-22. Are there exceptions to the trust rules under Medicaid?

There are three exceptions. The following trusts are exempt from the Medicaid trust rules:

- A trust established by a parent, grandparent, guardian, or court for the benefit of an individual who is disabled and under age 65, using the individual's own funds.

- A trust composed only of pension, Social Security, and other income of the individual, in states which make individuals eligible for institutional care under a special income level, but do not cover institutional care for the medically needy.

- A trust established by a disabled individual, parent, grandparent, guardian, or court for the disabled individual, using the individual's own funds, where the trust is made up of pooled funds and managed by a non-profit organization for the sole benefit of each individual included in the trust.

In all of the above instances, the trust must provide that the state receives any funds, up to the amount of Medicaid benefits paid on behalf of the individual, remaining in the trust when the individual dies.

A trust will not be counted as available to an individual where the state determines that counting the trust would work an undue hardship.

ESTATE RECOVERIES

H-23. Can a state recover nursing home and long-term care Medicaid expenses from the estate of a deceased Medicaid recipient?

States are required to recover the costs of nursing facility and other long-term care services furnished to a Medicaid beneficiary from the estate of the beneficiary unless undue hardship would result. The estate may include any real or personal property or other assets in which the beneficiary had any legal title or interest at the time of death, including the home. Different estate recovery provisions apply to individuals who purchase specified long-term care insurance policies in designated states.

According to the Centers for Medicare & Medicaid Services, "undue hardship" might exist when the estate subject to recovery is the sole income-producing asset of the survivors and the income is limited or is a homestead of modest value.

It is possible that a state may conclude that an undue hardship does not exist if the individual created the hardship by resorting to estate planning methods under which the individual divested assets in order to avoid estate recovery. A state may adopt a rebuttable presumption that if the individual obtained estate planning advice from legal counsel and followed this advice, the resulting financial situation would not qualify for an undue hardship waiver.

The estate recovery rules apply only to the estates of Medicaid beneficiaries dying on or after October 1, 1993, only to benefits paid on or after that date, and only for costs for a Medicaid recipient who was age 55 or older at the time the costs were incurred. Recovery of Medicaid costs cannot take place while the surviving spouse lives.

DISCRIMINATION

H-24. Does federal law protect Medicaid patients from discrimination by nursing homes?

There is no requirement that nursing homes participate in Medicaid. Nursing homes receive reimbursement for Medicaid patients but it is usually much lower than the rates nursing homes charge private-pay patients (those who use their own funds, insurance benefits, or a combination of the two). Most nursing homes participate in Medicaid, but the level of participation can vary. A nursing home can make all of its beds Medicaid beds, or it can have some Medicaid beds and some private-pay beds.

If a patient in a nursing home starts out paying privately, uses up all excess resources, and becomes eligible for Medicaid, the nursing home is prohibited by federal law from evicting the patient because the method of payment has changed from private payment to Medicaid. The patient can be evicted if he cannot pay the nursing home and is also ineligible for Medicaid.

The nursing home contract defines the rights and responsibilities of the nursing home and patient. There are limitations on certain contract provisions that affect Medicaid patients:

(1) A nursing home contract may not force the patient to give up the right to receive Medicare or Medicaid. A nursing home must counsel patients about the availability of these benefits.

(2) A nursing home contract may not force a relative or friend of the patient to guarantee payments in order to get the patient into the nursing home. A nursing home can require a person in charge of a potential resident's funds to commit those funds to the payment of nursing home bills.

(3) A nursing home cannot require a person or a person's family to pay more than the Medicaid rate in order to have a Medicaid-eligible person admitted to the nursing home.

MANAGED CARE

H-25. How has managed care changed the original Medicaid program?

A significant change to the original Medicaid program is the managed care concept. Under managed care systems, health maintenance organizations (HMOs), prepaid health plans (PHPs) or comparable entities agree to provide a specific set of services to Medicaid enrollees in return for fixed periodic payments per enrollee. Managed care programs seek to enhance access to quality care in a cost-effective manner. However, there are complexities in this, and waivers of certain parts of the Social Security Act are required. These waivers provide states with greater flexibility in the design and implementation of their Medicaid programs.

Section 1915(b) of the Social Security Act allows states to develop innovative health care delivery or reimbursement systems. Section 1115 of the Social Security Act allows statewide health care reform demonstrations for testing various methods of covering uninsured populations, and testing new delivery systems, without increasing costs.

Medicaid managed care programs are growing rapidly and several states have converted their entire Medicaid programs into managed care. Over 16 million Medicaid recipients are enrolled in Medicaid managed care programs–which is more than 50% of all Medicaid enrollees.

States can restrict choice by offering a choice between at least two managed care organizations or Primary Care Case Managers (PCCM), or at least one plan and one PCCM. States must permit individuals to change their enrollment for cause at any time, without cause within 90 days of notification of enrollment, and without cause at least every 12 months thereafter.

States may provide up to six months minimum enrollment that covers all managed care entities.

There are protection for Medicaid beneficiaries in managed care, including (1) assuring coverage of emergency services, (2) protection of enrollee-provider communications, (3) grievance procedures, (4) demonstration of adequate capacity and services, (5) protecting enrollees against liability for payment, and (6) antidiscrimination.

STATE LTC PARTNERSHIP PROGRAM

H-26. What is a "qualified state long-term care insurance partnership?"

Under the *Deficit Reduction Act of 2005 (DRA),* a qualified state long-term care insurance partnership is a state Medicaid plan amendment that provides for the disregard of assets or resources in an amount equal to the insurance benefit payments made to or on behalf of an individual who is a beneficiary under a qualifying long-term care (LTC) insurance policy.

A qualifying LTC partnership policy must meet the following requirements:

1. The policy covers an insured who was a resident of the state when coverage first became effective under the policy.

2. The policy is a tax-qualified LTC insurance policy issued not earlier than the effective date of the state LTC partnership program.

3. The policy must meet the standards contained in the 2000 NAIC Model LTC Policy Act and Regulations.

4. The policy must contain the following inflation protection provisions:

    a. Buyers younger than age 61—compound annual inflation protection
    b. Buyers ages 61-75—some level of inflation protection
    c. Buyers age 76 or older—no inflation protection required.

5. Agents selling the policy must receive appropriate training and demonstrate understanding of the policy.

6. The issuer of the policy must provide regular reports with information on policy benefits, claims, underwriting, terminations, and other information deemed appropriate.

7. The policy must not be subject to any state insurance mandates not applicable to all LTC insurance policies sold in the state.

The DRA lifted a 1993 ban on new state LTC partnership programs. Prior to the DRA, four states, California, Connecticut, Indiana, and New York, had LTC partnership programs adopted prior to the ban. The details of the existing programs vary with respect to policy requirements and the degree of asset protection provided to those purchasing the policies.

New state Medicaid plan amendments adopting LTC partnership programs may be effective October 1, 2007. As many as 20 states appear ready to implement state LTC partnership programs in 2007.

The DRA mandates standards for the uniform reciprocal recognition of LTC partnership policies under which benefits paid by such policies will be treated the same by all states with qualified state LTC insurance partnerships. A state with a LTC insurance partnership is subject to the standards unless the state formally elects to be exempt from such standards.

TABLE OF HOSPITAL INSURANCE (PART A)
Effective after January 1, 2007

Service	Benefit	Medicare Pays	A Person Pays
HOSPITALIZATION Semiprivate room and board, general nursing, and other hospital services and supplies.	First 60 days	All but $992	$992
	61st to 90th day	All but $248 a day	$248 a day
	91st to 150th day[1]	All but $496 a day	$496 a day
	Beyond 150 days	Nothing	All costs
SKILLED NURSING FACILITY CARE Semiprivate room and board, skilled nursing and rehabilitative services and other services and supplies.[2]	First 20 days	100% of approved amount	Nothing
	Additional 80 days	All but $124 a day	$124 a day
	Beyond 100 days	Nothing	All costs
POST-HOSPITAL HOME HEALTH CARE Part-time or intermittent skilled care, home health aid services, durable medical equipment and supplies and other services.	First 100 days in spell of illness	100% of approved amount; 80% of approved amount for durable medical equipment	Nothing for services; 20% of approved amount for for durable medical equipment
HOSPICE CARE Pain relief, symptom management and support services for the terminally ill.	For as long as the doctor certifies need	All but limited costs for outpatient drugs and inpatient respite care	Limited costs for outpatient drugs and inpatient respite care
BLOOD When furnished by a hospital or skilled nursing facility during covered stay.	Unlimited if medically necessary	All but first 3 pints per calendar year	For first 3 pints[3]

1. 60 Reserve days benefit may be used only once in a lifetime.
2. Neither Medicare nor private Medigap insurance will pay for most nursing home care.
3. Blood paid for or replaced under Part B of Medicare during the calendar year does not have to be paid for or replaced under Part A.

TABLE OF MEDICAL INSURANCE (PART B) BENEFITS
Effective after January 1, 2007

Services	Benefit	Medicare Pays	Patient Pay
MEDICAL EXPENSE Doctors' services, inpatient and outpatient medical and services surgical services and supplies, physical and speech therapy, diagnostic tests, durable medical equipment and other services.	Unlimited if medically necessary.	80% of approved amount (after $131 amount and limited deductible). Reduced to 50% for most outpatient mental health services.	$131 deductible,[1] plus 20% of approved charges above approved amount.[2]
CLINICAL LABORATORY SERVICES Blood tests, urinalyses, and more.	Unlimited if medically necessary.	Generally 100% of approved amount.	Nothing for services.
HOME HEALTH CARE Part-time or intermittent skilled care, home health aide services, durable medical equipment and supplies and other services.	Unlimited but covers only home health care not covered by Hospital Insurance (Part A).	100% of approved amount; 80% of approved amount for durable medical equipment.	Nothing for services; 20% of approved amount for durable medical equipment.
OUTPATIENT HOSPITAL TREATMENT Services for the diagnosis or treatment of illness or injury.	Unlimited if medically necessary.	Medicare payment to hospital based on hospital cost.	20% of whatever the hospital charges (after $131 deductible).[1]
BLOOD	Unlimited if medically necessary.	80% of approved amount (after $131 deductible and starting with 4th pint).	For first 3 pints plus 20% of approved amount for additional pints (after $131 deductible).[3]
AMBULATORY SURGICAL SERVICES	Unlimited if medically necessary.	80% of pre-determined amount (after $131 deductible).	$131 deductible, plus 20% of pre-determined amount.

1. Once a person has $131 of expense for covered services in 2007, the Part B deductible does not apply to any further covered services received for the rest of the year.
2. A person pays for charges higher than the amount approved by Medicare unless the doctor or supplier agrees to accept Medicare's approved amount as the total charge for services rendered.
3. Blood paid for or replaced under Part A of Medicare during the calendar year does not have to be paid for or replaced under Part B.

WHAT MEDICARE DOES NOT COVER

Some of these items can be covered by Medicare under certain conditions. See text for more detailed information on items covered under special conditions.

Acupuncture

Most chiropractic services

Cosmetic surgery (except after an accident)

Custodial care

Most dental care

Most prescription drugs and medicines taken at home (except through Medicare Part D)

Eyeglasses and eye examinations for prescribing, fitting, or changing eyeglasses

Foot care that is routine

Canadian or Mexican health care

Hearing aids and hearing examinations for prescribing, fitting, or changing hearing aids

Homemaker services

Meals delivered to the home

Naturopaths' services

Immunizations, except vaccinations against pneumococcal pneumonia, hepatitis B, or influenza virus; and immunizations required because of an injury or immediate risk of infection

Injections which can be self-administered

Nursing care on full-time basis in the home

Orthopedic shoes unless they are part of a leg brace and are included in the orthopedist's charge

Personal convenience items that the patient requests, such as a phone, radio, or television in the room at a hospital or skilled nursing facility

Physical examinations that are routine and tests directly related to such examinations

Private nurses

Private room

Services performed by immediate relatives or members of the patient's household

Services that are not reasonable and necessary

Services for which neither the patient nor another party on his behalf has a legal obligation to pay

Supportive devices for the feet

War claims occurring after the effective date of the patient's current Medicare coverage

Services payable by any of the following:

- Workers' Compensation (including black lung benefits)

- Liability or nofault insurance

- Employer group health plans for employees and their spouses

- Employer group health plans for people entitled to Medicare solely on the basis of end stage renal disease

- Another government program

EXAMPLE OF MEDICARE BENEFITS

Mr. Smith is 69 years old, retired, and covered by Hospital Insurance (Part A), Medical Insurance (Part B), and Prescription Drug Insurance (Part D). After suffering a heart attack at his home in January, 2007, he is taken to the hospital for surgery. Mr. Smith spends 15 days in the hospital and 7 days in a skilled nursing facility for therapy. When he returns home, he requires the services of a nurse and physical therapist for a short time to continue treatment.

	Total cost:	Mr. Smith pays:	Medicare pays:
Hospital bill: *(Patient pays the deductible amount)*	$3,500	$992	$2,508
Ambulance to hospital: *(Patient pays 20% plus amount higher than customary charge)*	$70	$14	$56
Surgeon: *(Patient pays $124 deductible and 20% of the remaining bill; Medicare pays 80% of the bill after the deductible)*	$2,000	$505	$1,495
Anesthesiologist: *(Patient pays 20%; Medicare pays 80%)*	$300	$60	$240
Skilled Nursing Facility: *(Patient pays nothing for first 20 days, then $119 a day for 80 days)*	$1,050	$0	$1,050
Home visits by nurse: *(Medicare pays for nurse required for medical reasons)*	$90	$0	$90
Home visits by physical therapist:	$80	$0	$80
Equipment rental (wheelchair): *(Patient pays 20%; Medicare pays 80%)*	$85	$17	$68
Prescription drugs at home: *(assuming standard $250 deductible)*	$200	$200	$0
Total Cost:	**$7,375**	**$1,788**	**$5,587**

FISCAL INTERMEDIARIES

Note: Fiscal intermediaries can answer questions about Hospital Insurance (Part A) bills and services, hospital care, skilled nursing care, and fraud. You may reach the fiscal intermediary for your state at 1-800-MEDICARE (1-800-633-4227).

State	Carrier
Alabama	Cahaba Government Benefits Administrators (GBA)
Alaska	Noridian Mutual Insurance Company
Arizona	Blue Cross Blue Shield of Arizona
Arkansas	Blue Cross Blue Shield of Arkansas
California	United Government Services
Colorado	TrailBlazer Health Enterprises, LLC
Connecticut	Empire Medicare Services
Delaware	Empire Medicare Services
Florida	First Coast Service Options, Inc.
Georgia	Blue Cross Blue Shield of Georgia
Hawaii	United Government Services
Idaho	Medicare Northwest
Illinois	Adminastar Federal, Inc.
Indiana	Adminastar Federal, Inc.
Iowa	Cahaba Government Benefits Administrators (GBA)
Kansas	Blue Cross Blue Shield of Kansas
Kentucky	Adminastar Federal, Inc.
Louisiana	Trispan Health Services
Maine	Associated Hospital Services
Maryland	Highmark Medicare Services
Massachusetts	Associated Hospital Services
Michigan	United Government Services
Minnesota	Noridian Mutual Insurance Company
Mississippi	Trispan Health Services
Missouri	Mutual of Omaha Insurance Companies
Montana	Blue Cross Blue Shield of Montana
Nebraska	Blue Cross Blue Shield of Nebraska
Nevada	Mutual of Omaha Insurance Companies
New Hampshire	Anthem Health Plans of New Hampshire-Vermont
New Jersey	Blue Cross Blue Shield of Tennessee
New Mexico	TrailBlazer Health Enterprises, LLC
New York	Empire Medicare Services
North Carolina	Palmetto Government Benefits Administrators (GBA)
North Dakota	Noridian Mutual Insurance Company
Ohio	Adminastar Federal, Inc.

State	Carrier
Oklahoma	Chisholm Administrative Services
Oregon	Medicare Northwest
Pennsylvania	Veritus Medicare Services
Rhode Island	Arkansas Blue Cross and Blue Shield
South Carolina	Palmetto Government Benefits Administrators (GBA)
South Dakota	Cahaba Government Benefits Administrators (GBA)
Tennessee	Blue Cross Blue Shield of Tennessee
Texas	TrailBlazer Health Enterprises, LLC
Utah	Medicare Northwest
Vermont	Anthem Health Plans of New Hampshire-Vermont
Virginia	United Government Services
Washington	Noridian Mutual Insurance Company
Washington D.C.	Highmark Medicare Services
West Virginia	United Government Services
Wisconsin	United Government Services
Wyoming	Blue Cross Blue Shield of Wyoming
American Samoa	United Government Services
Guam	United Government Services
Northern Mariana Islands	United Government Services
Puerto Rico	Cooperativa De Seguros De Vida (COSVI)
Virgin Islands	Cooperativa De Seguros De Vida (COSVI)

MEDICARE CARRIERS

Note: Carriers can answer questions about Medical Insurance (Part B). To reach any of the carriers, call 1-800-MEDICARE (1-800-633-4227). If you are entitled to Medicare under the Railroad Retirement system, send your Medical Insurance claims to Palmetto GBA, 1-800-833-4455.

State	Carrier
Alabama	Cahaba Government Benefits Administration (GBA)
Alaska	Noridian Mutual Insurance Company
Arizona	Noridian Mutual Insurance Company
Arkansas	Blue Cross/Blue Shield of Arkansas
California	National Heritage Insurance Company
Colorado	Noridian Mutual Insurance Company
Connecticut	First Coast Service Options, Inc.
Delaware	Trailblazer Health Enterprises, LLC
District of Columbia	Trailblazer Health Enterprises
Florida	First Coast Service Options, Inc.
Georgia	Cahaba Government Benefits Administrators (GBA)
Hawaii	Noridian Mutual Insurance Company
Idaho	CIGNA (Connecticut General Life Ins. Co)
Illinois	Wisconsin Physicians Service
Indiana	AdminaStar Federal, Inc.
Iowa	Noridian Mutual Insurance Company
Kansas	Blue Cross/Blue Shield of Kansas
Kentucky	AdminaStar Federal, Inc.
Louisiana	Blue Cross/Blue Shield of Arkansas
Maine	National Heritage Insurance Company
Maryland	TrailBlazer Health Enterprises, LLC
Massachusetts	National Heritage Insurance Company
Michigan	Wisconsin Physician Services
Minnesota	Wisconsin Physician Services
Mississippi	Cahaba Government Benefits Administration (GBA)
Missouri	Blue Cross/Blue Shield of Kansas (Western Missouri)
	Medicare Services of Missouri (Eastern Missouri)
Montana	Blue Cross/Blue Shield of Montana
Nebraska	Blue Cross/Blue Shield of Kansas
Nevada	Noridian Mutual Insurance Company
New Hampshire	National Heritage Insurance Company
New Jersey	Empire Medicare Services
New Mexico	Blue Cross/Blue Shield of Arkansas
New York	HealthNow of Upstate New York: Upstate
	Empire Medicare Services: Downstate
	Group Health, Inc. (GHI Medicare): Queens County

State	Carrier
North Carolina	CIGNA Medicare
North Dakota	Noridian Mutual Insurance Company
Ohio	Palmetto Government Benefits Administrators (GBA)
Oklahoma	Blue Cross/Blue Shield of Arkansas
Oregon	Noridian Mutual Insurance Company
Pennsylvania	HGS Administrators of Pennsylvania
Rhode Island	Blue Cross/Blue Shield of Arkansas
South Carolina	Palmetto Government Benefits Administrators (GBA)
South Dakota	Noridian Mutual Insurance Company
Tennessee	CIGNA Medicare
Texas	TrailBlazer Health Enterprises, LLC
Utah	Regence Blue Cross/Blue Shield of Utah
Vermont	National Heritage Insurance Company
Virginia	TrailBlazer Health Enterprises, LLC
Washington	Noridian Mutual Insurance Company
Washington, DC	Trailblazer Health Enterprises, LLC
West Virginia	Palmetto Government Benefits Administrators (GBA)
Wisconsin	Wisconsin Physician Service
Wyoming	Noridian Mutual Insurance Company
American Samoa	Noridian Mutual Insurance Company
Guam	Noridian Mutual Insurance Company
Northern Mariana Islands	Noridian Mutual Insurance Company
Puerto Rico	Triple-S, Inc.
Virgin Islands	Triple-S, Inc.

MEDICARE QUALITY IMPROVEMENT ORGANIZATIONS (QIOs)

*QIOs can answer questions about the quality of care and access to care in a Medicare-cer-
tified facility. QIOs cannot answer questions about a bill or about what Medicare covers.
For Part A or Part B billing or coverage questions, call your Part B carrier or your Part A
intermediary. See Appendix D. The toll-free or 800 numbers listed below, in many cases, can
be used only in the state or service areas indicated.*

State	Quality Improvement Organizations (QIOs)	Phone
Alabama	Alabama Quality Assurance Foundation, Inc.	1-800-760-4550
Alaska	Qualis Health	1-800-445-6941
Arizona	Health Services Advisory Group Inc.	1-800-359-9909
Arkansas	Arkansas Foundation for Medical Care, Inc.	1-800-272-5528
California	Lumetra	1-800-841-1602
Colorado	Colorado Foundation for Medical Care, Inc.	1-800-727-7086
Connecticut	Qualidigm	1-800-553-7590
Delaware	Quality Insights of Delaware	1-866-475-9669
District of Columbia	Delmarva Foundation for Medical Care, Inc.	1-800-645-0011
Florida	Florida Medical Quality Assurance, Inc.	1-800-844-0795
Georgia	Georgia Medical Care Foundation	1-800-979-7217
Hawaii	Mountain-Pacific Quality Health Foundation	1-800-524-6550
Idaho	Qualis Health	1-800-445-6941
Illinois	Illinois Foundation for Quality Health Care	1-800-647-8089
Indiana	HealthCare Excel, Inc.	1-800-288-1499
Iowa	Iowa Foundation for Medical Care, Inc.	1-800-752-7014
Kansas	Kansas Foundation for Medical Care, Inc.	1-800-766-3777
Kentucky	Health Care Excel, Inc.	1-800-288-1499
Louisiana	Louisiana Health Care Review, Inc.	1-800-433-4958
Maine	Northeast Health Care Quality Foundation	1-800-772-0151
Maryland	Delmarva Foundation for Medical Care	1-800-999-3362
Massachusetts	MassPro	1-800-334-6776*
Michigan	Michigan Peer Review Organization, Inc.	1-800-365-5899
Minnesota	Stratis Health	1-800-444-3423
Mississippi	Information and Quality Healthcare	1-800-844-0600
Missouri	Primaris	1-800-735-6776
Montana	Mountain-Pacific Quality Health Foundation	1-800-497-8232
Nebraska	Cimro of Nebraska	1-800-247-3004
Nevada	HealthInsight	1-800-748-6773
New Hampshire	Northeast Health Care Quality Foundation	1-800-772-0151
New Jersey	Peer Review Organization New Jersey, Inc.	1-800-624-4557*
New Mexico	New Mexico Medical Review Association	1-800-663-6351
New York	Island Peer Review Organization-PRO Inc.	1-800-331-7767
North Carolina	Medical Review of North Carolina	1-800-722-0468
North Dakota	North Dakota Health Care Review, Inc.	1-800-472-2902*
Ohio	Ohio KePRO,Inc.	1-800-589-7337
Oklahoma	Oklahoma Foundation for Medical Quality	1-800-522-3414
Oregon	Oregon Medical Professional Review Organization (OMPRO)	1-800-344-4354

State	Quality Improvement Organizations (QIOs)	Phone
Pennsylvania	Quality Insights of Pennsylvania	1-877-346-6180
Rhode Island	Rhode Island Quality Partners, Inc.	1-800-662-5028
South Carolina	Carolina Medical Review	1-800-922-3089*
South Dakota	South Dakota Foundation for Medical Care, Inc.	1-800-658-2285
Tennessee	Q Source	1-800-528-2655
Texas	Texas Medical Foundation	1-800-725-9216
Utah	HealthInsight	1-800-274-2290
Vermont	Northeast Health Care Quality Foundation	1-800-772-0151
Virginia	Virginia Health Quality Center	1-866-263-8402
Washington	Qualis Health	1-800-445-6941
West Virginia	West Virginia Medical Institute, Inc.	1-800-642-8686 x2266
Wisconsin	MetaStar	1-800-362-2320
Wyoming	Mountain Pacific Quality Health Foundation	1-800-497-8232
American Samoa	Mountain Pacific Quality Health Foundation	1-800-524-6550
Guam	Mountain Pacific Quality Health Foundation	1-800-524-6550
Northern Mariana Islands	Mountain Pacific Quality Health Foundation	1-800-524-6550
Puerto Rico	Quality Improvement Professional Research Organization	1-800-981-5062*
Virgin Islands	Virgin Islands Medical Institute	1-340-712-2444

* In-State Calls Only

DURABLE MEDICAL EQUIPMENT REGIONAL CARRIERS

To reach any of the carriers listed below call 1-800-MEDICARE (1-800-633-4227).

State	Regional Carrier
Alabama	Palmetto Government Benefits Administrators (GBA)
Alaska	CIGNA Medicare
Arizona	CIGNA Medicare
Arkansas	Palmetto Government Benefits Administrators (GBA)
California	CIGNA Medicare
Colorado	Palmetto Government Benefits Administrators (GBA)
Connecticut	HealthNow DMERC
Delaware	HealthNow DMERC
Florida	Palmetto Government Benefits Administrators (GBA)
Georgia	Palmetto Government Benefits Administrators (GBA)
Hawaii	CIGNA Medicare
Idaho	CIGNA Medicare
Illinois	AdminaStar Federal, Inc.
Indiana	AdminaStar Federal, Inc.
Iowa	CIGNA Medicare
Kansas	CIGNA Medicare
Kentucky	Palmetto Government Benefits Administrators (GBA)
Louisiana	Palmetto Government Benefits Administrators (GBA)
Maine	HealthNow DMERC
Maryland	Adminastar Federal, Inc.
Massachusetts	HealthNow DMERC
Michigan	AdminaStar Federal, Inc.
Minnesota	AdminaStar Federal, Inc.
Mississippi	Palmetto Government Benefits Administrators (GBA)
Missouri	CIGNA Medicare
Montana	CIGNA Medicare
Nebraska	CIGNA Medicare
Nevada	CIGNA Medicare
New Hampshire	HealthNow DMERC
New Jersey	HealthNow DMERC
New Mexico	Palmetto Government Benefits Administrators (GBA)
New York	HealthNow DMERC
North Carolina	Palmetto Government Benefits Administrators (GBA)
North Dakota	CIGNA Medicare
Ohio	AdminaStar Federal, Inc.
Oklahoma	Palmetto Government Benefits Administrators (GBA)
Oregon	CIGNA Medicare
Pennsylvania	HealthNow DMERC
Rhode Island	HealthNow DMERC
South Carolina	Palmetto Government Benefits Administrators (GBA)

State	Regional Carrier
South Dakota	CIGNA Medicare
Tennessee	Palmetto Government Benefits Administrators (GBA)
Texas	Palmetto Government Benefits Administrators (GBA)
Utah	CIGNA Medicare
Vermont	HealthNow DMERC
Virginia	AdminaStar Federal, Inc.
Washington	CIGNA Medicare
Washington, DC	AdminaStar Federal, Inc.
West Virginia	AdminaStar Federal, Inc.
Wisconsin	AdminaStar Federal, Inc.
Wyoming	CIGNA Medicare
American Samoa	CIGNA Medicare
Guam	CIGNA Medicare
Northern Mariana Islands	CIGNA Medicare
Puerto Rico	Palmetto Government Benefits Administrators (GBA)
Virgin Islands	Palmetto Government Benefits Administrators (GBA)

INSURANCE COUNSELING -GENERAL INFORMATION

In addition to insurance counseling, these offices
can answer questions about Medicare bills.

Alabama	1-800-243-5463	New Jersey	1-800-792-8820*
Alaska	1-800-478-6065*	New Mexico	1-800-432-2080*
Arizona	1-800-432-4040	New York	1-800-333-4114
Arkansas	1-800-224-6330	North Carolina	1-800-443-9354*
California	1-800-434-0222*	North Dakota	1-888-575-6611
Colorado	1-888-696-7213*	Ohio	1-800-686-1578
Connecticut	1-800-994-9422*	Oklahoma	1-800-763-2828*
Delaware	1-800-336-9500*	Oregon	1-800-722-4134*
Florida	1-800-963-5337	Pennsylvania	1-800-783-7067
Georgia	1-800-669-8387	Rhode Island	1-401-462-3000
Hawaii	1-888-875-9229	South Carolina	1-800-868-9095
Idaho	1-800-247-4422*	South Dakota	1-800-536-8197
Illinois	1-800-548-9034*	Tennessee	1-877-801-0044
Indiana	1-800-452-4800	Texas	1-800-252-9240
Iowa	1-800-351-4664	Utah	1-800-541-7735*
Kansas	1-800-860-5260	Vermont	1-800-642-5119*
Kentucky	1-877-293-7447	Virginia	1-800-552-3402
Louisiana	1-800-259-5301*	Washington	1-800-562-6900
Maine	1-800-262-2232*	Washington, DC	1-202-739-0668
Maryland	1-800-243-3425*	West Virginia	1-877-987-4463
Massachusetts	1-800-243-4636	Wisconsin	1-800-242-1060
Michigan	1-800-803-7174	Wyoming	1-800-856-4398
Minnesota	1-800-333-2433	American Samoa	1-888-875-9229
Mississippi	1-800-948-3090	Guam	1-888-875-9229
Missouri	1-800-390-3330	Northern Mariana Islands	1-888-875-9229
Montana	1-800-551-3191*	Puerto Rico	1-877-725-4300
Nebraska	1-800-234-7119	Virgin Islands	1-340-772-7368
Nevada	1-800-307-4444		
New Hampshire	1-800-852-3388*	* In-State Calls Only	

STATE AGENCIES ON AGING

Note: State agencies on aging can provide information and assistance on a variety of Medicare, insurance, and elder care issues.

Alabama
Department of Senior Services
RSA Plaza
770 Washington Avenue, Suite 470
Montgomery, AL 36130-1851
(800) 243-5463
(334) 242-5743

Alaska
Commission of Aging
Division of Senior Services
P.O. Box 110209
Juneau, AK 99811-0290
(907) 465-3250

Arizona
Department of Economic Security
Aging and Adult Administration
1789 West Jefferson Street, #950A
Phoenix, AZ 85007
(602) 542-4446

Arkansas
Division of Aging & Adult Services
Donaghey Plaza South, Suite 1417
P.O. Box 1417, Slot S-530
Little Rock, AR 72203-1437
(501) 682-2441

California
Department of Aging
1600 K Street
Sacramento, CA 95814
(916) 322-5290

Colorado
Division of Aging and Adult Services
Department of Human Services
1575 Sherman Street, Ground Floor
Denver, CO 80203-1714
(303) 866-2636

Connecticut
Division of Elderly Services
25 Sigourney Street, 10th Floor
Hartford, CT 06106-5033
(860) 424-5298

Delaware
Services for Aging & Adults with
Physical Disabilities
Dept. of Health & Social Services
1901 North DuPont Highway
New Castle, DE 19720
(800) 223-9074
(302) 577-4791

District of Columbia
Office on Aging
441 Fourth Street, NW, 9th Floor
Washington, DC 20001
(202) 724-5622

Florida
Department of Elder Affairs
4040 Esplande Way, Suite 152, Bldg. B
Tallahassee, FL 32399-7000
(800) 96ELDER
(850) 414-2000

Georgia
Division of Aging Services
Department of Human Resources
2 Peachtree Street N.E., 9th Floor
Atlanta, GA 30303-3142
(404) 657-5258

Hawaii
Executive Office on Aging
250 S. Hotel Street, Suite 109
Honolulu, HI 96813-2831
(808) 586-0100

Idaho
Commission on Aging
P.O. Box 83720
Boise, ID 83720-0007
(208) 334-3833

Illinois
Department on Aging
421 E. Capitol Avenue, #100
Springfield, IL 62701-1789
(800) 252-8966

Indiana
Bureau of Aging and
In-Home Services
402 W. Washington Street, #W454
P.O. Box 7083
Indianapolis, IN 46207-7083
(800) 545-7763
(317) 232-7020

Iowa
Department of Elder Affairs
200ð10th Street
3rd Floor
Des Moines, IA 50309-3709
(515) 242-3333

Kansas
Department on Aging
New England Bldg.
503 S Kansas Avenue
Topeka, KS 66603-3404
(785) 296-5222

Kentucky
Office of Aging Services
Cabinet for Family and Children
275 East Main Street
Frankfort, KY 40621
(502) 564-6930

Louisiana
Governor's Office of Elderly Affairs
P.O. Box 80374
Baton Rouge, LA 70806-0374
(225) 342-7100

Maine
Bureau of Elder & Adult Services
35 Anthony Avenue
State House, Station 11
Augusta, ME 04333
(207) 624-5335

Maryland
Department of Aging
301 W. Preston Street
Baltimore, MD 21201-2374
(410) 767-1100

Massachusetts
Executive Office of Elder Affairs
1 Ashburton Place, 5th Floor
Boston, MA 02108
(800) 882-2003
(617) 222-7451

Michigan
Office of Services to the Aging
611 W. Ottawa Street
N. Ottawa Tower, 3rd Floor
P.O. Box 30026
Lansing, MI 48909
(517) 373-8230

Minnesota
Board on Aging
444 Lafayette Road
St. Paul, MN 55155-3843
(651) 296-2770

Mississippi
Div. of Aging & Adult Services
750 N. State Street
Jackson, MS 39202
(800) 948-3090
(601) 359-4925

Missouri
Division of Senior Services
Dept. of Health & Senior Sciences
615 Howerton Court
P.O. Box 1337
Jefferson, MO 65109-1337
(800) 235-5503
(573) 751-3082

Montana
Division of Senior and Long-Term
Care/DPHHS
111 Sanders, Room 211
P.O. Box 4210
Helena, MT 59620
(800) 332-2272
(406) 444-4077

Nebraska
Division on Aging
P.O. Box 95044
1343 Main Street
Lincoln, NE 68509-5044
(800) 942-7830
(402) 471-2307

Nevada
Department of Human Resources
Division for Aging Services
State Mail Room Complex
3416 Goni Road, Bldg. D-132
Carson City, NV 89706
(775) 687-4210

New Hampshire
Division of Elderly & Adult Services
State Office Park South
129 Pleasant Street, Brown Bldg. #1
Concord, NH 03301
(603) 271-4680

New Jersey
Division of Senior Affairs
P.O. Box 807
Trenton, NJ 08625-0807
(800) 792-8820
(609) 943-3345

New Mexico
State Agency on Aging
La Villa Rivera Bldg.
228 East Palace Avenue, Ground Floor
Santa Fe, NM 87501
(800) 432-2080
(505) 827-7640

New York
State Office for the Aging
2 Empire State Plaza
Albany, NY 12223-1251
(800) 342-9871
(518) 474-7012

North Carolina
Division of Aging
2101 Mail Service Center
Raleigh, NC 27699-2101
(919) 733-3983

North Dakota
Department of Human Services
Aging Services Division
600 South 2nd Street, Suite 1C
Bismarck, ND 58504
(800) 755-8521
(701) 328-8910

Ohio
Department of Aging
50 W. Broad Street, 9th Floor
Columbus, OH 43215-5928
(800) 282-1206
(614) 466-5500

Oklahoma
Department of Human Services
Aging Services Division
312 N.E. 28th Street
Oklahoma City, OK 73125
(405) 521-2327

Oregon
Seniors & People with Disabilities
500 Summer Street, N.E., 2nd Floor
Salem, OR 97310-1015
(800) 232-3020
(503) 945-5811

Pennsylvania
Department of Aging
Forum Place
555 Walnut Street, 5th Floor
Harrisburg, PA 17101-1919
(717) 783-1550

Puerto Rico
Governor's Office of Elderly Affairs
Call Box 50063
Old San Juan Station, PR 00902
(787) 721-5710

Rhode Island
Department of Elderly Affairs
160 Pine Street
Providence, RI 02903-3708
(401) 462-0500

South Carolina
Office of Senior & LTC Services
P.O. Box 8206
Columbia, SC 29202-8206
(803) 898-2513

South Dakota
Office of Adult Services & Aging
700 Governor's Drive
Pierre, SD 57501-2291
(605) 773-3656

Tennessee
Commission on Aging & Disability
Andrew Jackson Bldg., 9th Floor
500 Deaderick Street
Nashville, TN 37243-0860
(615) 741-2056

Texas
Department of Aging & Disability Services
701 West 51st Street
Austin, TX 78751
(512) 438-3011

Utah
Division of Aging & Adult Services
120 North 200 West
Salt Lake City, UT 84145-0500
(801) 538-3910

Vermont
Dept. of Aging and Disabilities
103 S. Main Street
Waterbury, VT 05671-2301
(802) 241-2400

Virginia
Department for the Aging
1610 Forest Avenue, Suite 100
Richmond, VA 23229
(800) 552-3402
(804) 662-9333

Washington
Aging & Adult Services Administration
Dept. of Social & Health Services
P.O. Box 45050
Olympia, WA 98504-5600
(360) 725-2310

West Virginia
Bureau of Senior Services
Holly Grove, Bldg. 10
1900 Kanawha Blvd. East
Charleston, WV 25305
(304) 558-3317

Wisconsin
Bureau of Aging & Long Term Care Resources
1 West Wilson Street, Room 450
Madison, WI 53707
(800) 242-1060
(608) 266-2536

Wyoming
Division on Aging
6101 Yellowstone Road, Suite 259B
Cheyenne, WY 82002-0710
(800) 442-2766
(307) 777-7986

CENTERS FOR MEDICARE & MEDICAID SERVICES

Regional Office	Customer Service	States Served
Atlanta	404-562-7500	AL,FL,GA,KY,MS,NC,SC,TN
Boston	617-565-1232	CT,ME,MA,NH,RI,VT
Chicago	312-353-7180	IL,IN,MI,MN,OH,WI
Dallas	214-767-6401	AR,LA,NM,OK,TX
Denver	303-844-2111	CO,MT,ND,SD,UT,WY
Kansas City	816-426-2866	IA,KS,MO,NE
New York	212-264-3657	NJ,NY,PR,VI
Philadelphia	215-861-4226	DE,DC,MD,PA,VA,WV
San Francisco	415-744-3602	AZ,AS,CA,GU,HI,MP,NV
Seattle	206-615-2354	AK,ID,OR,WA

MEDICARE ADVANTAGE PPO REGIONS

CMS has established 26 regions for the Medicare Advantage Regional Preferred Provider Organizations authorized by the Medicare Prescription Drug, Improvement, and Modernization Act of 2003. (See SECTION D for more information.)

State	MA PPO Region	State	MA PPO Region
Alabama	10	Montana	19
Alaska	26	Nebraska	19
Arizona	21	Nevada	22
Arkansas	15	New Hampshire	1
California	24	New Jersey	4
Colorado	20	New Mexico	20
Connecticut	2	New York	3
Delaware	5	North Carolina	7
District Of Columbia	5	North Dakota	19
Florida	9	Ohio	12
Georgia	8	Oklahoma	18
Hawaii	25	Oregon	23
Idaho	23	Pennsylvania	6
Illinois	14	Rhode Island	2
Indiana	13	South Carolina	8
Iowa	19	South Dakota	19
Kansas	18	Tennessee	10
Kentucky	13	Texas	17
Louisiana	16	Utah	23
Maine	1	Vermont	2
Maryland	5	Virginia	7
Massachusetts	2	Washington	23
Michigan	11	West Virginia	6
Minnesota	19	Wisconsin	14
Mississippi	16	Wyoming	19
Missouri	15		

Region	State	Medicare Beneficiaries in Region	Medicare Beneficiaries in State
1	Maine	422,515	235,804
	New Hampshire		186,711
2	Connecticut	1,805,085	536,258
	Massachusetts		995,597
	Rhode Island		176,688
	Vermont		96,542
3	New York	2,845,450	2,845,450
4	New Jersey	1,255,829	1,255,829

Region	State	Medicare Beneficiaries in Region	Medicare Beneficiaries in State
5	Delaware	901,259	125,231
	District Of Columbia		77,195
	Maryland		698,833
6	Pennsylvania	2,527,088	2,167,299
	West Virginia		359,789
7	North Carolina	2,239,963	1,258,190
	Virginia		981,773
8	Georgia	1,655,581	1,019,216
	South Carolina		636,365
9	Florida	3,041,852	3,041,852
10	Alabama	1,663,097	750,732
	Tennessee		912,365
11	Michigan	1,501,197	1,501,197
12	Ohio	1,784,284	1,784,284
13	Indiana	1,588,640	910,980
	Kentucky		677,660
14	Illinois	2,555,008	1,720,335
	Wisconsin		834,673
15	Arkansas	1,389,193	471,368
	Missouri		917,825
16	Louisiana	1,107,824	650,510
	Mississippi		457,314
17	Texas	2,504,912	2,504,912
18	Kansas	947,170	405,801
	Oklahoma		541,369
19	Iowa	1,913,827	496,059
	Minnesota		702,052
	Montana		148,409
	Nebraska		264,491
	North Dakota		105,887
	South Dakota		125,645
	Wyoming		71,284

Region	State	Medicare Beneficiaries in Region	Medicare Beneficiaries in State
20	Colorado New Mexico	778,442	516,005 262,437
21	Arizona	769,443	769,443
22	Nevada	291,959	291,959
23	Idaho Oregon Utah Washington	1,764,310	186,976 535,276 230,812 811,246
24	California	4,257,579	4,257,579
25	Hawaii	182,651	182,651
26	Alaska	51,198	51,198

Beneficiary data from Centers for Medicare & Medicaid Services MA PPO fact sheet published in September 2005.

Do You Know What You're Missing?

**Year After Year, Rules Change.
Strategies Change.
Even Solar Systems Change.**

See reverse for de[tails]

RETURN POLICY

100% Satisfaction Guaranteed

National Underwriter is confident you'll be pleased with our powerful resources. Your total satisfaction is guaranteed 100% of the time. If your expectations are not met or a product is damaged in shipping, contact us within 30 days from the invoice date for immediate resolution. Your purchase is refundable in the form of your original payment. Special rules apply for certain items:

1) CE Exams, Electronic Products, CD-ROMs, and Shipping & Handling are not refundable.

2) Subscriptions to newspapers, periodicals and loose-leaf services may be cancelled within 30 days from delivery of a first installment. Loose-leaf services must be returned for a full refund.

SHIPPING & HANDLING

Order Total		S&H
$0	to $39.99	$6.95
$40.00	to $79.99	$8.95
$80.00	to $124.99	$11.95
$125.00	to $199.99	$15.95
$200.00	to $249.99	$18.95

Add shipping and handling charges to all orders as indicated. If your order exceeds total amount listed in chart, or for overseas rates, call 1-800-543-0874. **Any order of 10 or more items or $250 and over will be billed for shipping by actual weight, plus a handling fee.** Any discounts do not apply to Shipping & Handling.

QTY	ITEM DESCRIPTION	PRODUCT #	RETAIL 1-9	SALE PRICE 10 OR MORE	TOTAL PRICE
	2007 Tax Facts Complete Power Combo²	TFBPC07	$164.90	CALL	
	2007 Tax Facts on Insurance & Employee Benefits	2920007	$47.95	$43.16 (10+)	
	2007 Field Guide to Estate Planning, Business Planning, & EB	1790007	$44.95	$40.46 (10+)	
	2007 Tax Facts on Investments	2930007	$47.95	$43.16 (10+)	
	2007 Field Guide to Financial Planning	1780007	$44.95	$40.46 (10+)	
	2007 Benefits Facts	603007	$59.95	$53.96 (10+)	
	2007 ERISA Facts	1170007	$44.95	$40.46 (10+)	
	2007 Social Security & Medicare Kit	586007	$49.90	$44.91 (10+)	
	2007 Social Security Source Book	2860007	$27.95	$25.16 (10+)	
	2007 All About Medicare	1460007	$21.95	$19.76 (10+)	
	2007 Social Security Slide-O-Scope & Planner Set (set consists of 5)	2810007	$27.95	$25.16 (10+)	
	2007 Medicare Planner Set (set consists of 5)	1710007	$13.95	$12.56 (10+)	

Promo Code: BCARD

Offer Ends 10/30/07.

Discounts are based on a minimum purchase of the same title/product number. If you do not meet the minimum quantity to qualify for the printed discount, you will be invoiced at the retail price.

☐ Invoice Me   ☐ Call Me

Sales Tax: Residents of CA, CT, DC, FL, GA, IL, KS, KY, MI, NJ, NY, OH, PA, TX and WA must add appropriate sales tax

SUBTOTAL $ _____

Shipping & Handling (see chart) $ _____

ORDER TOTAL $ _____

Company _____ Title _____

Name _____

Phone ( ) _____ E-mail _____

Address _____ Fax ( ) _____